❧ Armfuls of Time

✿ Armfuls of Time

The Psychological Experience of the Child
with a Life-Threatening Illness

Barbara M. Sourkes, Ph.D.

University of Pittsburgh Press
Pittsburgh and London

Published by the University of Pittsburgh Press, Pittsburgh, Pa. 15260
Copyright © 1995, University of Pittsburgh Press
All rights reserved
Manufactured in the United States of America
Printed on acid-free paper

The epigraph on page vi is reprinted with permission of Scribner, an imprint of
Simon & Schuster, from *Vesper Sparrows* by Deborah Digges. Copyright © 1986
by Deborah Digges.

Color plates xxvii and xxviii are reprinted with permission of Patricia Lynch-
Ordynec and the publisher of Humane Medicine 9 (January 1993).

LIBRARY OF CONGRESS CATALOGING-IN-PUBLICATION DATA
Sourkes, Barbara M.
    Armfuls of time : the psychological experience of the child with a
life-threatening illness / Barbara M. Sourkes.
      p. cm.
    Includes bibliographical references.
    ISBN 0-8229-3888-x (acid-free paper).—ISBN 0-8229-5565-2
(pbk.: acid-free paper)
    1. Critically ill children—Psychology.   2. Critically ill children—
Mental health.   3. Child psychotherapy—Case studies.   4. Tumors in children—
Psychological aspects.   I. Title.
RJ370.S68   1995
618.92'001'9–dc20   95–8667
                                             CIP

A CIP catalogue record for this book is available from the British Library.

Eurospan, London

for my parents

I want to say don't worry, I can save myself,
I can find my way into a future where
sunlight recovers its losses . . .

—*Deborah Digges*

✢ Contents

❧ Acknowledgments

Grateful acknowledgment is made to the following individuals and foundations; all have contributed to *Armfuls of Time*.

Frederick A. Hetzel, director of the University of Pittsburgh Press, has been a sustaining friend. His wisdom, encouragement, and humor have accompanied me through the writing of both my books. Catherine Marshall is a most sensitive editor.

I wish to express my thanks to Philip Hallen, president of the Maurice Falk Medical Fund, and Rosalyn Markovitz, who led me to the United Jewish Federation in Pittsburgh; Arthur H. Jaffe; and the University of Pittsburgh Medical Center.

David G. Nathan, Robert A. Stranahan Professor of Pediatrics, Harvard Medical School, extended loyalty and support to me. He also helped me to obtain the David Abraham Fellowship at the Dana-Farber Cancer Institute. Nancy Upp Potter, Dana-Farber Cancer Institute, and Martha E. Cassin, Massachusetts General Hospital, have been devoted friends to me and to this book. I am also grateful to Kurt J. Isselbacher, director of the Massachusetts General Hospital Cancer Center.

Harvey J. Cohen, chairman of the Department of Pediatrics, Stanford University, and Margaret C. Kiely, professor of Psychology, Université de Montréal, provided invaluable consultation and perspective on the manuscript. Thanks to Nancy R. Treves for her clinical material; and, with Pamela M. Ryan, when both were at the

x Acknowledgments

Children's Hospital in Boston, for the photography in "My Life Is Feelings." My friends and colleagues at the Dana-Farber Cancer Institute and the Children's Hospital in Boston, and now at the Montreal Children's Hospital, have contributed to the richness and enjoyment of my work over the years.

My most profound gratitude is to all the children who are portrayed in *Armfuls of Time*. It is a privilege to have entered their lives. I wish to make particular acknowledgment to the following children and their families: Jennifer Cause, Karen Josephson, Jonathan Nason, and Richard (Ricky) Segelbaum. Thanks to the family of Amy Potter for her two poems, and to the families of Jonathan (Jay) Hager and Damian Lynch for their drawings. The voices and images of all the children express the essence of *Armfuls of Time*.

✽ Prologue

I just wish that I had armfuls of time.

In the longing expressed by a four-year-old child, the abstraction of time becomes palpable and real. *Armfuls of Time* examines the psychological experience of the child with a life-threatening illness. From the physical reality of illness and treatment, to its impact on daily life, to the psychic horizons of awareness, the child is irreversibly changed by the diagnosis. How he or she *lives* with life-threatening illness forms the theme of this book.

A life-threatening illness is a disease that may possibly end in death. A prolonged period of living with the illness may thus precede death, if it occurs. Through medical advances, many diseases of childhood that were once of short duration and uniformly fatal have become chronic in nature and do not necessarily result in death. While in many instances recovery and even cure may be achieved, the child and family nonetheless experience the reverberations of anticipatory grief. Whether or not the threat of death transforms into actuality, profound uncertainty prevails.

This book focuses on the child with cancer. However, the clinical issues that I address are relevant for other chronic or life-threatening diseases characterized by intermittent hospitalizations and disruptions. A common denominator among the disorders is their relentless and insistent presence. Such diseases include AIDS, cystic fibrosis, sickle cell anemia, renal disease, and congenital heart disease. In these illnesses the threat of separation and death is no longer the only focus, although it is still omnipresent.

Armfuls of Time concerns the child who is in, or near the time of, active treatment; that is, who is still intimate with the physical rigors of the illness itself. It is not about long-term survivorship, although future-oriented issues are certainly alluded to in the immediacy of the experience. I focus on the child between the ages of three and twelve—I do not venture into the experience of the adolescent—and, while the family provides the framework for the discussion, my specific lens remains on the child-who-is-the-patient.

I have worked with children for almost twenty years, at the Dana-Farber Cancer Institute and the Children's Hospital in Boston, and currently at the Montreal Children's Hospital. With few exceptions (noted in the text), all the psychotherapeutic material that I describe in this book is based on my own clinical work, documented in detailed notes that I took during, or immediately after, psychotherapy sessions with the children. (Many of the sessions with Ricky were tape-recorded; these dialogues are the actual transcripts.)

I have integrated the experiences of many children; four, with whom I worked intensively, are named, and their words weave throughout the text. They are (in the order they appear in the book): Ricky, Karen, Jonathan, and Jenny. I knew Jenny from the time of her diagnosis at age nine until age twelve, and I have culled material from this three-year period. I followed the other three children from a later point in their illness, each for about one year. Ricky and Jonathan were approximately six years old, and Karen was about nine. I also include two poems by twelve-year-old Amy.

The children's art provides a visual counterpoint to the text.

Drawing is a familiar task for this age group and serves as a powerful means of expression. It often goes beyond the verbal level, enabling the emergence of profound realizations.

Armfuls of Time may be seen as a companion to my first book, *The Deepening Shade,* where I synthesized the psychology of life-threatening illness within the overarching framework of time. The pervasive theme of that book was that all individuals, regardless of age, share in a common struggle as the illness unfolds. The reader was led, cognitively and emotionally, into the experience of those who live with uncertainty.

This book opens with "Psychotherapy," a chapter that both conceptually and clinically provides the context for the therapeutic work. The remaining chapters examine the child's experience from his or her perspective. "Illness and Treatment" describes the immediate impact of the diagnosis on the child and the physical onslaught that he or she must endure in the struggle to recover. I consider bone marrow transplantation specifically, since it is an extremely stressful procedure that is becoming more common in pediatrics. In this chapter I also discuss the milestone of elective cessation of treatment and the ever present threat of relapse. "Impact on Normal Life" moves outward from the core of the illness and treatment into the realm of family, school, and peers. How does the child reenter these spheres after the diagnosis and find a new semblance of normalcy? "Facets of Awareness" concerns the child's intrapsychic experience of the illness. He or she may talk directly about its life-threatening potential, or allusively through references to time. Dreams and emergent spiritual beliefs also attest to the awareness. "Anticipatory Grief" examines the omnipresence of threatened separation in emotional terms of loss of relationships. "The Dying Child" focuses on imminent death. It is important to note that, with the exception of this last chapter, the book focuses on the child *living* with illness, rather than dying of it.

Armfuls of Time highlights the child's adaptation to life-threatening illness with the acknowledgment of potential sources of vulnerability. These pages reveal resilience and courage, and it is in this spirit that the book begins.

❧ Armfuls of Time

❧ Psychotherapy

I felt much better because I knew that I had somebody to talk to
all the time. Every boy needs a psychologist! To see his feelings!
(Ricky)[1]

If every hair on your head fell out, don't you think you'd need a
talking doctor? *(eight-year-old boy)*

Psychotherapy with the child who has a life-threatening illness is
profound and poignant, and it powerfully attests to the struggle toward survival. Within its framework, the child seeks to reintegrate
the shattered facets of his or her life. Through words, drawings, and
play, the child conveys the experience of living with the ever present
threat of loss and transforms the essence of his or her reality into expression.

Most children enter psychotherapy because of the stress engendered by the illness, rather than more general intrapsychic or interpersonal concerns. From a psychological point of view, the majority
of the children are well adjusted. Psychopathology is the exception,
not the rule. In *The Spiritual Life of Children,* the child psychiatrist
Robert Coles remembers advice offered by Erich Lindemann, a psychoanalyst, during the polio epidemic of the 1950s. Parallels to the
child with cancer and other life-threatening illnesses are evident.

These are young people who suddenly have become quite a bit older;
they are facing possible death, or serious limitation of their lives; and

they will naturally stop and think about life, rather than just live it from day to day. A lot of what they say will be reflective—and you might respond in kind. It would be a mistake, I think, to emphasize unduly a psychiatric point of view. If there is serious psychopathology, you will respond to it, of course; but if those children want to cry with you, and be disappointed with you, and wonder with you where their God is, then you can be there for them.[2]

Lindemann thus reminds the therapist to "bear witness" to the child's extraordinary situation, and to respond within the context of that reality.

THE CONCEPTUAL FRAMEWORK

The concept of psychic trauma lends itself to understanding the experience of life-threatening illness in childhood. Lenore Terr, a child psychiatrist, offers the following definition: "'Psychic trauma' occurs when a sudden, unexpected, overwhelmingly intense emotional blow or a series of blows assaults the person from outside. Traumatic events are external, but they quickly become incorporated into the mind. A person probably will not become fully traumatized unless he or she feels utterly helpless during the event or events."[3]

This description certainly relates to the overwhelming sense of loss of control experienced by the seriously ill child: the shock of diagnosis, the indelible imprint of the sustained assault on the body and psyche, and the uncertainty of the outcome. Whereas malevolence of intent characterizes many forms of trauma (such as abuse or kidnapping), the culprit in life-threatening illness is the inexplicable, impersonal randomness of fate.

Donald Winnicott, the first British pediatrician to become a psychoanalyst, wrote extensively about the developmental processes of childhood and their implications for psychotherapy. He defined trauma as "an impingement from the environment and from the individual's reaction to the environment that occurs prior to the individual's development of mechanisms that make the unpredictable predictable."[4]

While life-threatening illness does not literally originate in the environment, its devastating impact on the child more than qualifies it as trauma. In fact, the illness goes beyond what Winnicott referred to as "unthinkable anxieties" in its *actual* threat of death.[5] Winnicott further stressed the importance for the young child of the "presentation of the world in small doses . . . the preservation of a certain amount of illusion—an avoidance of too sudden insistence on the reality principle."[6] The child with a life-threatening illness stands unshielded from pain, terror, and the ultimate threat of loss of life. In this sense, it is no exaggeration to state that he or she loses a critical aspect of childhood in the moment of diagnosis.

Play enables the seriously ill child to "reenter" childhood. It is for this reason that the playrooms in the hospital and clinic are such crucial settings, operating as the emotional hub of the treatment center for the child. They grant the child respite from the harshness of the immediate environment. In *Road Song,* a memoir of growing up in Alaska, Natalie Kusz describes her experience of the life-threatening injuries she sustained at age seven after being attacked by a dog. She illuminates the importance of the playroom in the hospital.

There was a playroom in the children's wing, a wide room full of light, with colored walls and furniture, and carpets on the floor. A wooden kitchen held the corner alongside our infirmary, and my friends and I passed many hours as families, cooking pudding for our dolls before they were due in therapy. Most of the dolls had amputated arms and legs, or had lost their hair to chemotherapy, and when we put on our doctors' clothes, we taught them to walk with prostheses, changing their dressings with sterile gloves. We had school tables and many books, and an ant farm by the window so we could care for something alive. . . . Within [this] playroom, some of us were handicapped, but not disabled, and in time we were each taught to prove this for ourselves.[7]

In child psychotherapy, play is the crucial vehicle of communication. Winnicott differentiated between "to *play at* (thus coping with) rather than *to be in* the frightening fantasy."[8] While the child with a life-threatening illness is always confronting reality rather than fantasy (or, reality in addition to fantasy), Winnicott's distinction highlights a definitive function of play. He further stressed that enjoyment of the play is an a priori condition of entering into the depth of the psychotherapeutic process. For the seriously ill child whose very existence is suffused with gravity, such pleasure is intrinsically valuable.

The overwhelming nature of the illness cannot be approached by reality alone. Paradoxically, the illusion afforded by play is what allows reality to be integrated. Through play, the child can advance and retreat, draw near and pull away from the intense core. These tentative forays allow the child to contain and master the experience. Illusion is not to be construed as avoidance; on the contrary, play is the essence of a child's expression. Furthermore, illusion is translucent, if not transparent, and thus reality shines through for both the child and the therapist even when not addressed directly by either.

Disturbances in play occur primarily in children with developmental disorders, severe psychopathology, or deprivation. However, the trauma of life-threatening illness can extinguish—at least temporarily—some children's capacity for play, or erode its range of expression into rigid patterns. Within the context of psychotherapy, a certain restoration is marked when the child's play reveals its former vitality.

The therapist's willingness and ability to enter into the play are of utmost importance. Shared imaginative play enables the child to confront the realities of life and death. The psychotherapy session described here is a cameo of such collaboration.

Ricky had recently acquired a rubber axe. He pretended that there was a whale swimming alongside the bed. (The whale was invisible). Ricky was vehemently trying to kill the whale with the axe, because one of his stuffed animals, Wally Skubeedoo Walrus, wanted to eat it for supper. Ricky kept asking: "Is the whale dead yet?" The therapist would look over the side of the bed and report that it was still swimming or blowing bubbles. Finally, the therapist suggested that Ricky check whether the whale was alive or dead. Ricky said: "I'll listen to his heart." He pretended to use a stethoscope and said: "Th-thump, th-thump. . . . He's still alive because his heart is beating." The therapist commented: "If the whale's heart is beating, then he isn't dead yet." Ricky looked startled and said: "But I don't want him to be dead." It appeared that Ricky had not associated the fact of killing the whale with the whale being dead. Ricky leaned over the side of the bed to ask the whale how he was feeling. The whale answered (in the therapist's voice) that his back was sore from all the hitting, but that he would like to be Ricky's friend. Ricky agreed, and named him "Mr. Whaley Whale Friend." He then threw down his axe in disgust. The therapist wondered aloud how Ricky might use his axe in a more constructive way. Ricky decided that when he raised his axe, it would mean that all his stuffed animals must pay attention. Ricky then asked his animals the following riddle: What did the big axe say to the little axe? Triumphant answer: Don't kill whales!

Inextricably linked with play is the child's use of symbolic language. The words themselves (not simply the thematic content) often reveal images that are idiosyncratic to a particular child and consistent over time. They provide windows into his or her experience.

Images of cold (winter, ice water, ice age) were associated with fear and death in Ricky's stories and play. The dichotomous "up-down" was his indicator of whether or not things were going well. For example, "my heart was down" was his description of a medical crisis from which he had just emerged. An eight-year-old girl relied on this polarity as well. One day in the clinic, she informed the therapist: "Playing is up, but school is down." For both children, "up-down" may have been associated originally with blood counts or mood; it then generalized in their usage.

The therapist's knowledge of normal development is essential in evaluating the impact of life-threatening illness on the child. Cognitive, affective, and social perspectives intersect at every juncture. The child's cognitive comprehension enables emotional mastery, while, reciprocally, the lived experience allows for conceptualization that would ordinarily lie beyond his or her grasp. Social factors (interpersonal and cultural) provide the framework, either facilitative or hindering, for the child's adaptation.

In complementary ways, the developmental theories of Jean Piaget and Erik Erikson provide a context for understanding the child's experience. Piaget's theory of cognition emphasizes the active role of the child in discovering and constructing reality, evolving from a sensorimotor approach, through stages of concrete reasoning, to the capacity for abstraction. An ever shifting dynamic equilibrium exists between the processes of assimilation of and accommodation to the exigencies of the external world.[9] Erikson describes psychosocial "crises" that the child must negotiate in the formation of his or her sense of self and in relation to others (trust versus mistrust, autonomy versus shame and doubt, initiative versus guilt, and industry versus inferiority).[10] The child's passage through both Piaget's and Erikson's developmental stages is challenged to the utmost in the presence of serious illness.

Although most psychological problems of the child with a life-threatening illness may be categorized as adjustment reactions, more severe psychopathology can emerge. This is especially true in the child with preexistent vulnerabilities or when there is a prior psychiatric history in the child or a family member. While it is important not to overemphasize pathology in the child, there is also a risk in minimizing or not recognizing it. Furthermore, any psychological response, however benign initially, can freeze into a traumatic reaction under sustained stress. Thus, the therapist must be able to assess the severity of symptoms, particularly in terms of intensity and duration, relative to the child's current reality. For example, if reactive depression or anxiety (which resolve relatively easily) develop into major clinical disorders, more intensive psychotherapy and psychotropic medication may be required. Disordered eating that originates as a secondary effect of the illness and treatment can develop into an eating disorder unto itself or indicate significant depression. Difficult behaviors in a child may result in his or her becoming a "behavior problem" in settings beyond the medical center. Such clinical situations require careful differentiation by the therapist.

In addition to the knowledge of normal development and psychopathology, the therapist must be well informed of medical facts and their implications. The latter requirement grounds the therapist in the reality of the child's life situation and thus is crucial for the psychotherapy to be effective.

A psychodynamic conceptualization provides the framework for the author's work with the child with a life-threatening illness. However, as Terr points out: "Even though the therapy of childhood trauma is often modeled upon psychoanalytic principles, the treatment will work out quite differently."[11] Each therapist must find a pathway to the child that is congruent with his or her own training, experience, feelings, and attitudes. The willingness to improvise, and to be alert to the spontaneous, contribute to the vitality of the psychotherapeutic process. The psychic and physical demands on the child translate into enormous challenges for the therapist.[12]

THE THERAPIST'S ROLE

What does the child understand of the therapist's role and of the psychotherapy process itself? It is important that simple, nonthreatening explanations be offered to the child. Terms like "the talking doctor" provide a functional description that clearly distinguish the therapist from other professionals on the medical team. The anxiety about seeing a therapist can be allayed by explaining that all children who are ill have worries and that the therapist can help with these problems. The concept of confidentiality, or privacy, should be introduced early, with a definition of its meaning and its boundaries. Over time, even if not articulated, the child comes to understand the therapist's role in his or her care.

The therapist explained to Ricky that as "a talking doctor," her role was to talk and play with children, rather than to examine and give medicine. "What do you think of that?" she asked. Ricky responded enthusiastically: "I think that's great!" Two months later, he recommended to Poly Polar Bear, one of his stuffed animals: "Talk to Dr. Sourkes —that's what she's here for." As the therapist left the room that day, Ricky asked tentatively, trying out the word for the first time: "Are you a psy-chol-o-gist?"

The therapist came to the hospital room of a nine-year-old boy who had just been diagnosed. He talked animatedly about the current world series in baseball. When he asked the therapist's opinion as to the outcome, she admitted: "I really don't know much about sports." He looked at her quizzically and retorted: "What *do* you know about—hospitals?"

On one of her clinic visits, Karen's physician asked her how she was feeling. She answered: "Medically I'm fine, but psychologically I'm not so fine, but I'll discuss that with my psychologist."

As important as it is for the child to know what the therapist can provide, the limits of the role must also be delineated. The issue of expectations often emerges once the psychotherapeutic process is well underway.

Ricky was playing with Sealy Seal, one of his stuffed animals, when the therapist came into his room. In Sealy Seal's voice, he addressed the therapist:

Ricky: Hello, Dr. Sourkes. Would you buy me some fresh fish tomorrow?
Therapist: I don't think so, Sealy Seal. That's not my job around here. Do you know what my job is?
Ricky: Of course! Playing with Ricky!
Therapist: That's right, Sealy Seal. And talking with Ricky and answering questions.
Ricky: [impatiently, in his regular voice] Just deliver him some fried fish!
Therapist: I can't promise him that.

The definition of the therapist's role relates directly to the therapeutic alliance and transference. For the child who lives under threat, the establishment of a secure therapeutic alliance is an intervention in and of itself. Transference, the feelings that the child projects on the therapist, develops in a parallel process. While transference is always a crucial vehicle for the exploration of feelings, the therapist must be vigilant to contain its intensity. The psychotherapeutic relationship itself should not take up an inordinate amount of "space" in the child's limited psychic reserves. Rather, the transference can fuel the child's available energy for relationships and activities outside the boundaries of the illness.

PSYCHOTHERAPEUTIC TECHNIQUES

Psychotherapy with the seriously ill child demands that unstructured associative communication be combined with highly focused interventions. The author has found the following psychotherapeutic techniques to be particularly evocative: the therapeutic stuffed animal, lists, letter-writing, the incomplete sentence story, creation of a book, and the therapist's monologue. Art techniques include the mandala, the change-in-family drawing, and the "scariest" image.

Given the specific focus on the emotional reverberations of the illness, the therapist can be highly selective in choosing the materials for the psychotherapy. Absolute essentials include one or more stuffed animals or dolls, art materials, and an array of medical supplies related to the child's treatment. Most children are not intrigued by a plastic doctor's kit; it is too simplistic and innocent in light of their experience. In contrast, the opportunity to handle the real medical objects in a nonthreatening context facilitates desensitization and mastery. The portability of these essential supplies extends the range of the therapist's office—if the child is hospitalized, the therapist can "bring" his or her office to the child. The familiarity of the objects facilitates the transfer of the psychotherapy to a different setting.

A second tier of toys includes a dollhouse and family figurines, play hospital settings, and selected picture books related to illness and hospitalization in childhood. The classic *Curious George Goes to the Hospital* is enduringly popular, especially in combination with a Curious George stuffed animal.[13] Beyond these core supplies, each therapist develops his or her own selection to enable the child's creative expression in the psychotherapeutic setting.

The Therapeutic Stuffed Animal

Many of the children mentioned in this book have meaningfully involved a stuffed animal in their psychotherapy. This is not a coincidence; rather, the author has made the use of an animal pivotal in her work. The evolution and significance of this technique are described here; the clinical vignettes throughout the book provide the elaboration.

The author's recognition of the profound value of integrating a stuffed animal *in a sustained way* in psychotherapy began with Ricky. He arrived for every hospitalization with a menagerie of animals, each named (Poly Polar Bear, Wally Skubeedoo Walrus, Myrtle Dog, and so on) and designated as his son, daughter, nephew, niece, or wife. Occasionally these established relationships would change. Of a total "cast of characters" of thirty, he brought a different selection of about eight animals on each admission. He would assemble the animals on his bed and play with them for hours. Their initiation into the psychotherapeutic process occurred quite spontaneously one day when Ricky and the therapist were discussing another child's death.

Therapist: Ricky, look at Poly Polar Bear. He looks very sad and he is not playing.
Ricky: Is he sad because Johnny died?
Therapist: I guess so. What shall we do?
Ricky: He should play, because playing makes time go faster.

From that moment on, Poly Polar Bear became an important

spokesperson to reflect feelings, particularly sadness. Ricky made this link explicit when he stated: "When Poly is sad, I am sad."

After Ricky's death, his parents gave Poly Polar Bear to the therapist. She placed him on a shelf in her office, among a few other stuffed animals. Several months later, Karen noticed Poly. She picked him up and said: "This polar bear looks very sad. What's his name?" By the next session, Karen announced: "I give Poly feelings." Two weeks later she declared to the child life specialist in the hospital: "I'm one of the few people who understands Poly." Poly Polar Bear went on to play a crucial role in her psychotherapy, even becoming the subject of a book entitled *My Life Is Feelings* (see the appendix).

The animal may be introduced into the psychotherapeutic process simply as one of the therapist's toys or with a more focused agenda. In the latter instance, the therapist draws attention to the animal and discloses that it is being treated for the same illness as the child. Most children are intrigued by this connection (even if skeptical) and question the therapist about the animal's experiences. Through this commonality, an alliance between the child and animal is formed. For a child who is receptive to this form of play, the identification with the animal and the projective process do not take long to establish.

With the exception of Karen, who continued to use Poly Polar Bear's original name (provided spontaneously by the therapist), the other children in the book named the therapeutic animal themselves. Thus, Jonathan called a teddy bear "Walnut Bear" because its label indicated nutshells in the stuffing. Jenny named a squirrel "Nutty," while another child referred to it as "Freddy." (When more than one child uses the same animal, the therapist must take great care not to mix up the names!) The therapist brought the squirrel to her first meeting with a four-year-old boy in the hospital. He immediately reached over and kissed it! The therapist began to phrase questions to him through the squirrel: "Squirrel wants to know whether you like to be in the hospital? [No.] Squirrel wants to know whether you feel sad? [Yes.]" The boy then asked the squirrel: "Did you ever throw up? Did you ever have an operation?" At the end of this session, he named the squirrel "Kiss." A few weeks later, the boy arrived for a clinic appointment carrying a bag of peanuts for Kiss. His first question to the therapist was whether Kiss had missed him while he was at nursery school.

By naming the animal, the child gives it a distinct identity and simultaneously asserts a definite proprietary claim. Interestingly, in addition to the chosen name, many children use a combination of either their own or the therapist's family name for the animal. Thus, each of Ricky's animals also had his family's surname. The four-year-old boy gave Kiss both his own and the therapist's family names ("Kiss _____ Sourkes"). Jenny added "Nutty Sourkes" onto her file in the therapist's office, after her own name.

Although using one of the child's own animals is certainly not precluded, he or she is often reluctant to involve it extensively in the psychotherapy. Furthermore, the animal already carries its own history and associations and thus has less power of projection. For these reasons, it is often better to leave the child's animal as a safe object of comfort, with only peripheral involvement in the therapeutic process. Even with Ricky—whose network of animals was unique— the *therapist's* singling out and sustaining Poly Polar Bear as the one therapeutic animal was the critical intervention. In her work with children other than Ricky, the author has provided the therapeutic animal.

What is the significance of the therapeutic stuffed animal to the child and thus to the process? In certain ways, the animal resembles Winnicott's "transitional object," a special possession adopted by the infant or young child that becomes vitally real and important.[14] The child "assumes rights" over this object, which is notable for withstanding intense positive and negative emotion. The transitional object functions as a bridge between the child's inner psyche and his or her recognition of the outer world. Within the psychotherapy, the stuffed animal "lives" in the relationship between the child and the therapist. The animal belongs to the therapist; yet by naming it and sharing identical experiences, the child comes to "own" it. The therapist's animal becomes vital to the child and (in the child's mind) he or she to the animal, thus indirectly strengthening the therapeutic alliance. Through the authority of actual ownership, the therapist can impute feelings or comment more assertively than if the animal were the child's.

The child may find ways to integrate the therapeutic animal with his or her own animals. For example, Karen "invited" three of her animals from home to the birthday party she held for Poly Polar Bear. The four-year-old boy brought Kermit the Frog to a session "to meet" Kiss the Squirrel. The specialness of the therapeutic animal is thus acknowledged, without diminishing the role of the other animals in the child's outside life.

Lists

A technique that enables the child to focus on illness-related problems without undue stress is the compilation of a list entitled: "All the things I don't like about being sick," or "about treatment," or "about the hospital."[15] With the title at the top of a page, the child either writes or dictates the list. The therapist elicits specific details. Issues identified and prioritized by the child become targets for intervention, whether through discussion and play or through relaxation and hypnosis techniques. The child feels a sense of mastery in the amelioration of problems or change in attitude over time. Topics most often addressed include: medical procedures, nausea, hair loss, hospitalization, school and peer problems, and general worry about medical status.

A seven-year-old girl made this list of all the things she didn't like about being sick: "(1) The kids in school ask me questions that I don't know the answers to. (2) I don't know how to read. (3) I feel hungry but I just can't eat because I throw up. After it feels sour in my throat. (4) I don't like the bone marrows and the spinal taps. They hurt too much. Too many needles. The numbing medicine is the worst part because it feels like your leg is going to sleep. You feel like you want to move it and you can't because they're holding you down. It's not fun. (5) I don't like coming to the clinic."

An eight-year-old boy dictated a list of what he didn't like about being in the hospital: "(1) The food stinks. (2) You don't get to see your pets. (3) There's nothing to do. (4) Needles hurt. (5) Throwing up all the time. (6) You miss your parents."

Keeping a parallel list for a stuffed animal or doll to which the child is attached infuses an element of play into the process.

Karen listed the most difficult aspects of a long hospitalization. For herself, she wrote: "(1) Getting a blood transfusion. When the blood is cold, it feels like a knife cutting you. (2) Being awakened during the night for vital signs. (3) Hearing little kids scream." As for Poly Polar Bear: "(1) He hates needles—but he was fortunate not to have any this time. (2) He is afraid of spinal taps, so when he came in with me, he didn't watch. (3) Mostly he's scared of the abominable snowman."

The child can use lists effectively to formulate questions ahead of time for the caregivers, particularly at a critical juncture in treatment. The questions are often unpredictable, affording clues into the child's concerns and priorities. Medical issues may be overshadowed by a host of questions related to day-to-day living. In the child's ability to pose the questions, he or she asserts a degree of control. (See p. 72 for an example of a "question list.")

Letter-writing

Writing letters within the session can be an interesting and playful alternate route of communication. The letters may be between the child and the therapist, or involve a stuffed animal. The therapist can often phrase questions or observations through the letter that the child receives with less threat than if directly confronted. Even if the child does not reply to the questions, he or she is made aware that the therapist "knows."

The following correspondence among Jenny, Nutty the Squirrel, and the therapist illustrates the use of letter-writing within sessions. Jenny had been somewhat hesitant about trying relaxation techniques, and thus the therapist used Nutty to encourage her. While Jenny never actually described the nightmares mentioned in the letters, the acknowledgment of their existence seemed to be an effective intervention in and of itself. Jenny's spelling is left intact.

Dear Nutty,
How are you doing? Did you do anything new? Have you found any good nuts to eat? Today you have to have a finger stick. I hope you have been behaving yourself. Have you been watching your diet? Do you like hot chocolate? I do. NO bone maroe OR Spinel Tap today! Study your letters and numbers. Love you very, very, very, very much. Love, Jenny.

Dear Jenny,
This is the first time I've ever gotten a letter. Squirrels don't usually get mail, so I am very lucky! I haven't done anything new since I last

saw you. I have been eating well, but I haven't had any chocolate lately.
I'm so glad that I don't have to have a bone marrow or spinal tap today.
They scare me because they hurt. But Dr. Sourkes told me about some
special relaxation that she is going to teach me where I can use my
imagination to help myself. I hope that you will learn it with me so
that we won't get too nervous when we have procedures! I love you too.
I promise to study my letters and numbers before I see you next time.
It's lucky that Dr. Sourkes can help me type. Love, Nutty. [written by
therapist]

Three weeks later:

Dear Nutty,
    How are you? I hope that you took good care of Jenny last week
when you visited her in the hospital. I know that she felt very sick and
was glad to have you there. You and Jenny and I have to practice our
relaxation, and make a tape. Jenny's mother is a little bit worried about
all the nightmares Jenny has been having lately. . . . Do you know what
they have been about? And do you have any suggestions on how to
help them go away so that she is not scared at night? Please answer my
letter right away. Love, your friend, Dr. Sourkes.

Dear Nutty,
    Have you practiced your number and letter facts? I gave Curious
George an IV. You and I have to get going on the relaxashon texnecks.
Love, Jenny.

Dear Jenny,
    I can't wait to practice our relaxation techniques together! And to
get a special tape from Dr. Sourkes! About those nightmares, Jenny. . . .
Sometimes when I have been very sick like you were last week, I have
them too. But they go away after awhile, and you can feel safe knowing
that I am your special friend who understands. Love, Nutty. [written by
therapist]

Dear Jenny,

I'm GLAD your night mars went away. Sign out till next week. LOVE, Nutty. [written by Jenny]

One month later (a letter to Nutty written jointly by Jenny and the therapist):

Dear Nutty,

I love my new house. And I've got A LOT of new friends. How are you doing? Do you like your new place in the office? The kids are very nice at school. [Jenny]

Jenny's mother said that Jenny hasn't felt like using her relaxation tape lately. That's okay—she can just use it when she wants to when she is at home. But I hope that you will encourage her to practice it before she goes into the hospital, because she did SO WELL last time. You would have been very proud. Even though her spinal tap still bothered her, she handled it much better. So, don't forget to practice before procedures! [therapist]

This is your numbers test $2 \times 8 = 6 + 9 = \$2.35 + \$4.65 =$ Do well—you will need it. Love, Jenny and Dr. Sourkes. [Jenny]

Incomplete Sentence Story

This technique is particularly useful with the child who does not yet write and who enjoys dictating his or her thoughts. The therapist proposes that they tell a story together and provides the beginning of each sentence, as well as occasional questions. The topics relate to issues currently relevant to the child. A main character for whom the child chooses a name enhances the story's projective quality. In the following example, Ricky's contributions are italicized:

Once upon a time there was a little dog named . . . *Max.* Max was in an isolation room and . . . *he was Dr. Sourkes's dog.* What Max liked best about the isolation room was . . . *that he could have dog biscuit soup—but only low-bacteria kind.* What he didn't like was that . . . *it was far away from home in Detroit* [Ricky's home]. *It was in Chicago.* Was Max alone? *No. Dr. Sourkes stayed there with him. Even his brothers and sisters and father and mother. It was raining and winter in Chicago. It was snowing there in spring and summer and fall.* One night, Max was in the room all by himself . . . *Wrong! Only one person was with him— his brother.* Max didn't feel well. . . . *He had a headache. The doctor came in and put an icebag on his head and that's what they did to me! It was all water by morning.* Did Max and the doctor talk? *No, because Max had a toothache and they took his IV out and took him to the dentist.* Max need-ed white cells . . . *like me! Daddy's vein blew yesterday.* Who gives Max his white cells? *His brothers and sisters and cousins and friends and moth-er and father—even his grandma and grandpa. I miss my grandma all the time and I think about the food I'm going to eat all the time when I get home.*

A week later, Ricky spontaneously continued the story of Max: "Max has been in isolation for four months. No—make that four years." When the therapist commented that that was a very long time, Ricky responded: "But you were there with him! Max called yesterday. He told me that he had to get platelets. Max is going to stay as long as I am. Maybe he might have to stay for a very long time. All his blood is going up!" The therapist then asked Ricky whether he had a message for Max. Ricky said: "Tell him I love him. I will send him six puppy dogs on Friday."

Creation of a Book

The child is often intrigued by the idea of writing (or dictating) and illustrating a book about his or her experience of the illness. As with many interventions, the book becomes an intermediary be-tween the child and the therapist, allowing more threatening materi-al to be discussed than might be possible directly. Such books range from the simple to the sophisticated and may deal either implicitly or explicitly with the illness. Details such as choosing a title, decorating the cover, and stapling the pages together are all important in the child's experience of a book that is complete unto itself. Jonathan's *The Namey-Name Book,* its content metaphorical, was composed within one session (see color plates XVIII–XXIII). In contrast, *My Life Is Feelings* became the essence of Karen's psychotherapy over a three-month period (see the appendix).

Given Karen's attachment to, and identification with, Poly Polar Bear, the therapist suggested that she write a book about him. Karen enthusiastically agreed, adding that the book could be for other children who are sick. Because her psychotherapy had focused on articulating and labeling emotions, Karen and the therapist decided that the book would be about Poly Polar Bear's feelings. Thus the title evolved: *My Life Is Feelings.* The book was created in stages. First, a list of Poly's feelings was generated. Photographs were then taken of Poly to depict each feeling. Karen and the therapist decided to work on one feeling in each session. After discussion of the issues, based upon both Karen's and Poly's experience, she would write the text. Early in the process, Karen had decided that the book should have its own publication date. On that day, she and Poly Polar Bear presented copies of the book to her family, physician, and therapist. While *My Life Is Feelings* served to integrate Karen's individual experience, it synthesizes many issues common to the child living with a life-threatening illness.

The Therapist's Monologue

In this technique, the therapist articulates what he or she believes the child is thinking or feeling, without any demand on expression. The monologue should be used extremely selectively, reserved for those situations where the therapist judges that the child simply *cannot* form the words on his or her own, yet is longing to be understood. These are times when the child is withdrawn; either too exhausted physically to talk or paralyzed by intense vulnerability. Unspeakable terrors are often holding him or her hostage. However, through the therapist's musings, the child hears the actual "unsayable" words framed into a context, feels understood, and thus experiences reconnection and relief. These therapeutic effects are often manifested dramatically through words, body language, or behavior.

The therapist may talk about the child directly, allude in more general terms to how "some children feel," or use a therapeutic stuffed animal as the subject. If another adult is present, he or she can be involved adjunctively in the monologue. The therapist should speak slowly, calmly, and repetitively, not emphasizing any one point over another. He or she should proceed from peripheral to core issues in successive approximations, allowing the child time to absorb each level. The child need only listen, or answer yes or no to questions. Often the yes is signaled simply through sustained attention.

A four-year-old girl had refused to speak to anyone for days during a difficult hospitalization. Prior to the onset of the silence, she had cried about missing her baby sister. After greeting the girl and receiving no response, the therapist began talking about "kids being angry and sad." The child listened intently as the therapist covered such topics as: "Kids are angry that they have so many things done to them when they are in the hospital. . . . They are mad because the needles hurt. . . . Kids hate to be disturbed all the time when they are trying to sleep. . . . They are sad that they can't be at home with their families. . . . Kids are sad when they miss their sisters." The therapist continued, now involving the child life specialist who had just come into the room:

Therapist: I bet that she misses her sister too. Do you know her sister's name?
Specialist: No, I don't know her name.
Therapist: Me neither.
Child: [yelling] IT'S LINDA.

The child became teary at this point, and she allowed the therapist and child life specialist to sit closer to her and engage her in play with her teddy bear.

ART TECHNIQUES

Art therapy can be a powerful tool to facilitate the child's expression and integration of complex experiences.[16] Structured art techniques allow the therapist to pose questions earlier in the process and with more specificity than might be done through verbal means alone. Three structured techniques developed by the author are described below; examples of spontaneous drawings can be found in subsequent chapters.

Mandala

The mandala—a graphic symbolic pattern or design in the form of a circle—originated in Eastern religions. Jung believed that a mandala could mirror the state of the inner self.[17] The mandala is used in art therapy today, when a therapist asks a person to fill in a blank circle to reflect "how you are feeling now." The steps in a more structured version of this projective technique include: definition of topic, guided visualization, set of feelings, color-feeling match, proportion of color-feelings, and discussion of the completed mandala.

The therapist *defines a topic* around which the mandala will be focused. An example would be: "How I felt when I heard that I had cancer" (see color plates I and II). The therapist begins by providing the child with a brief *guided visualization*:

Close your eyes and think about the day you were diagnosed with cancer. Remember where you were [hospital, doctor's office, clinic], who was with you, who told you the diagnosis, what words were used. Remember how you felt. You may open your eyes.

The visualization sets the stage for the concrete task that follows:

Now I am going to give you the names of feelings which other children have told me they felt when they heard the diagnosis. I want you to think about each feeling and see if it fits for you.

The therapist then presents a *set of feelings* that are commonly attributed to the experience. Each feeling should be written on a separate file card and arranged randomly on the table to avoid the order bias of a vertical list. The feelings might include: shocked, scared, sad, angry, lonely, hopeful. A category called "other feelings" should also be included. It is best to limit the number of feelings to a maximum of eight. The therapist then gives the child a set of markers or crayons and a sheet of paper with the outline of a circle on it:

Now, *choose a color to match each feeling.* I want you to color in a part of the circle for each feeling. If the feeling was big, then make it a big part of the circle; if it was small, color in a small area [*proportion*]. You may use the same color for more than one feeling as long as you label it clearly. If you had other feelings that I have not mentioned, put them in. When you are all finished, we can *talk about the feelings and the colors* you have chosen.

Because the mandala requires little time and minimal exertion or coordination, it can be used even with a child who is very ill. Most children find the technique nonthreatening and enjoyable, and they often express relief at having an array of feelings already articulated for them. Interpretation of the mandala is based on the child's choice of feelings, colors, proportions, order, overall design, and verbal associations. At its simplest, the mandala is a tool for facilitating expression; at its most complex, it is powerful in its symbolism and depth.

Change-in-Family Drawing

The Kinetic Family Drawing is a widely used art therapy technique.[18] The child is asked to draw a picture of the entire family and to show each member engaged in an activity. The drawing is then analyzed for the child's perception of his or her position within the family and the nature of the family relationships. If the child is hesitant to engage in this task, he or she can be encouraged simply to draw stick figures. Although the richness of individual representation is lost, the dynamics of the family system nonetheless emerge. The author has added another step to this technique. After the child has completed the basic family portrait, the therapist asks: "What changed in your family after you got sick? Show the change in your drawing, either in picture or in words" (see figures 3 and 4 in chapter 2). The responses to this simple question are often dramatic and can be used for any "before and after" situation.

Scariest Image

The therapist asks: "Think of the *scariest* experience, thought, feeling, or dream that you have had since you became ill. Draw it." Through this technique, the therapist invites the child to bring out the extreme fear, often the very image that he or she is most afraid to express. The drawings tend to focus on medical procedures, being alone, and death (see, for example, figures 15, 21, 29 in chapters 2 and 3). They often represent a blend of actual and imagined experiences.

Drawings enable the emergence of profound disclosures. Although these art techniques are simple to administer, they evoke complex and powerful responses. The therapist must be prepared for the conscious and unconscious material that the pictures reveal.

WORK WITH PARENTS

With the intrusion of the illness, the relationship between child and parents organizes around the pivot of potential loss. Thus, it is critical that the therapist not intercede as a divisive wedge between them. From the outset, an ongoing alliance between the child's therapist and the parents diminishes this threat and optimizes the outcome of the work. Such collaboration is a sine qua non of the process. Because the parents must sustain the therapeutic work in the child's day-to-day encounters with both physical and emotional stresses, their role cannot be underestimated. Terr, in her work with traumatized children, comes to similar conclusions.

It is almost impossible for a [therapist] to treat a child without providing some access to parents . . . who participate in the child's life. Parents need the reassurance of visiting the [therapist]. They need to know what the [therapist] is doing, to know how the child is faring in treatment, and to know what specific plans for the child they must put into operation themselves. Once the [therapist] is out of the picture, the family has to take over. Much of the therapeutic process consists of preparing for that time.[19]

In working with both sides of the parent-child dyad, the therapist becomes aware of emerging developments and concerns and of issues that should be addressed with the child. Since the boundaries of confidentiality are more permeable than in traditional psychotherapy, the therapist must explain to the child how information will be shared with the parents. Most children express relief at knowing of this communication and even feel an increased security, provided that their own relationship with the therapist remains intact.

The mother of a four-year-old boy often wrote the therapist a letter between sessions. She included anything significant that had arisen since the last appointment. The following is an example of such a letter: "(1) He cries that we don't let him do anything because he's sick. That's not true. We only put restrictions on him when he's got low counts. (2) He hates being sick and says he 'hates the whole world.' We all feel like that at times. (3) Now when he's upset he doesn't come to me for comfort. He goes to his room, closes the door and wants to be left alone. If I go in, it's 'get out' or 'leave me alone.' He's shutting me out. WHY??? (4) He's still asking about death. He wants to know if we'll cry when he dies. We're trying to answer him honestly. (5) He's more demanding than ever. I tell him: 'Get it yourself. You're not sick—your blood is.' (6) Discipline is still a problem." The mother would either mail the letter to arrive before a scheduled session or bring it with her. If the therapist met with the boy prior to seeing his parents, he would hand the letter to the therapist to read while he took out his toys. He considered "being the mailman" a part of his routine. The mother's communications alerted the therapist to issues that needed to be addressed in the session.

As long as a ten-year-old boy met separately with his therapist, he did not protest the therapist's meetings or telephone contact with his parents. He knew that these discussions focused on his coping with the illness. Interestingly, when his mother was upset one day about matters unrelated to his illness, the boy suggested that she talk to the *other* psychologist in the clinic.[20]

The child's sense that the therapist "belongs" primarily to him or her can be easily enhanced. For example, the child can initially "show" the parents the therapist's office and supplies, thus establishing a sense of territoriality. When the child arrives eager to begin an appointment, the therapist need meet only briefly with the parents; more detailed discussion can follow the child's session.

If two therapists are involved with the family, the child's therapist must carve out a route of access to the parents that is acceptable to everyone. This includes: having the parents' therapist alert him or her to significant developments; keeping the parents' therapist well informed of the child's progress; and scheduling occasional joint meetings to enable direct contact among all the adults.

The range and depth of work with parents can vary greatly, from a concentrated focus on child-management issues (as is discussed here), to more traditional psychotherapy of the individual or the couple. Whatever the framework, the parents' reactions to the child's illness and the impact on their marriage and family are the organizing themes. In their own extreme state, the parents must find the strength to care for their even more vulnerable child: a formidable challenge to psychic resilience. Over time, the therapist's support becomes a resource from which the parents can draw.

The therapist facilitates and empowers the parents' interaction with medical professionals. Through rehearsal and modeling, the parents learn to formulate questions more effectively and to increase their confidence in communicating their concerns. In many instances, as a member of the interdisciplinary team, the therapist is present for these discussions. In addition, and with the parents' consent, the therapist may share selective aspects of the therapeutic material that bear directly on the care of the child. Such information includes: the child and family's present emotional status; any current stressors outside the illness; implications for their ability to cope at the moment; and recommendations for management. Content that does not contribute to these categories is generally best left unsaid. In promoting the parents' interactions with the medical team, and through these direct communications, the therapist plays a pivotal role in the integration of the child's total care.

The therapist can also enhance the parents' understanding of, and competence with, their child. By sharpening their observation and listening skills, they become associates in the therapeutic process. At the outset, the parents tend to report conversations or incidents involving the child, seeking the therapist's consultation as to their significance and management. Through the psychotherapeutic process, they gradually move toward offering their own interpretation and suggestions. In keeping the parents informed about the direction of the child's therapy, their grasp of his or her experience is further deepened. In this context, it is important that the therapist explain the importance of any animal or object to which the child has become attached during the psychotherapy. For example, once the parents understand the role of a stuffed animal as "alter ego," that animal can be incorporated into their conversations with the child. This inclusion provides the child and parents an additional route of communication with one another and extends the boundaries of the therapy into daily life. Relaxation techniques are valuable for the parents to learn with the child, so that eventually they can help him or her through medical procedures or at home. *Any* means of intervention that the therapist can provide for the parents to use with the child is an antidote to their helplessness.

Family therapy can play a pivotal role in sustaining, strengthening, and repairing family resources. The profound and enduring impact of the child's illness on the family is addressed within this context. In no way does family therapy preclude or contradict the individual psychotherapy with the child. Rather, it affirms the family unit as a whole, and provides a framework for its healing.

✌ Illness and Treatment

> *Therapist:* If you could choose one word to describe the time since your diagnosis, what would it be?
>
> *Child:* PAIN.[1]

Life-threatening illness is filled with hardship and terror for the child on both a physical and emotional level. Its ravages are an entity to be reckoned with on an ongoing basis, not a psychic abstraction. From the moment of diagnosis, the illness wends a perilous course; the unknown lies ahead like an uncharted chasm, without boundaries or guides.

DIAGNOSIS

When I heard that I had leukemia, I turned pale with *shock*. That's why I chose yellow—it's a pale color. *Scared* is red—for blood. I was scared of needles, of seeing all the doctors, of what was going to happen to me. I was *MAD* [black] about a lot of things: staying in the hospital, taking medicines, bone marrows, spinal taps, ivs, being awakened in the middle of the night. I was *sad* [purple] that I didn't have my toys and that I was missing out on everything. I chose blue for *lonely* because I was crying about not being at home and not being able to go outside. Green is for *hope:* getting better, going home, eating food from home, and seeing my friends (color plate i).[2]

This description of a mandala by an eight-year-old boy captures the immediacy of the response to the diagnosis of a life-threatening illness. He articulates the shock; the fear of everything from concrete medical procedures to the sudden possibility of an altered future ("what was going to happen to me"); the constellation of sadness, grief, and loneliness of separation; and his absence from normal life. Accompanying all these feelings is a forthright statement of hope.

In another description of the reaction to diagnosis, an eleven-year-old girl reflected:

Red is for *shock*—it's like coming to a stoplight, or like being hit by a bolt of lightning. *Anger* is black because it's a very, very dark feeling. You feel *scared* all the time of what is going to happen to you [purple]. *Alone* is blue, for tears, because you are so *sad*. I chose yellow for *hope*, because it's a sunny color, with a lot of light. *Helpless* [green] is little in my drawing, because that's just how you feel—tiny and scared. I made *confused* a mixture of all the colors together. You're just confused about everything going on and how this could all be happening to you (color plate II).

Other feelings cited by children include pain, terror, embarrassment, and shame. All these words attest to the overwhelming onslaught of new and frightening experiences that must be quickly assimilated. Such is the "irreversibly altered reality" into which the child is catapulted by the diagnosis.[3] Regardless of which aspects of life may appear unchanged, in fact, nothing is the same. The diagnosis thus stands as a dividing line, a marker of "before and after." The child, who garners security from predictability, and whose sense of time and timing is not yet well anchored, is thrust into a world of uncertain contingencies. The profundity of the disruption is daunting even to imagine.

It is the parents who are first told the diagnosis. Candor, reassurance, and realistic hope are essential components of its communication.[4] Information must initially be presented as clearly and simply as possible despite the urgent pressure to begin treatment. Parents who are reeling from the shock can absorb only a limited amount of information at the outset, and much repetition may be necessary over the next few days and weeks. This careful approach is an essential foundation, because almost immediately after diagnosis, the parents must sign the informed consent document for their child's treatment. In addition to describing the treatment that the child will undergo, it includes every known side effect, complication, and risk of the protocol. While intended as a factual document, its emotional impact on the parents cannot be underestimated. It stands as written confirmation of the child's vulnerability and of their own responsibility in all that lies ahead.

Much attention has been devoted to the impact of telling versus not telling the child the diagnosis and prognosis. The protective stance of the past stated that disclosure to the child would cause increased anxiety and fear. Over the last two decades, however, a shift toward open communication has been evident. To shield the child from the truth may only heighten anxiety and cause the child to feel isolated, lonely, and unsure about whom to trust. While the diagnosis is an event in time, "telling" is a process over time: "The time of diagnosis is a very stressful time for all involved.... Decisions made at this point ... are not etched in stone and are remade several times as the disease and treatment progresses."[5]

This caution tempers the pressure—or zeal—felt by some caregivers to "tell all immediately." How to inform the child of the diagnosis should be decided by the parents in consultation with the staff, thereby establishing a crucial alliance from the outset. The parents' design for the disclosure must be carefully heeded: it is they who know the child best and can gauge his or her resilience in absorbing the news. Furthermore, it is the parents who will see the child through every phase of the illness. The individual child's competence and vulnerability serve as the context for decisions regarding disclosure. Considerations about what or how much to tell include: the child's age, cognitive and emotional maturity, family structure and functioning, cultural background, and history of loss. In communication with the life-threatened child at any juncture, "the truth is not a principle nor a duty nor a rule. The truth is an atmosphere of exchange, of listening, and of respect for the child and his needs. The truth is a state."[6] The precedent for a climate that enables such honest interchange is created from the time of diagnosis.

Fluidity is a hallmark of the child's response to diagnosis: different emotions surge to the forefront or recede into the background at different times. In the following examples, one child reacts aggressively to the intrusion of the illness, while another's reaction is quieter and more pensive.

A three-year-old boy had frequent tantrums in which he screamed: "I hate being sick—I hate everyone." Or, without any apparent trigger, he would kick his dog, offering "I feel mean and angry" as his explanation. Then he would cry bitterly. On a brief hospitalization soon after his diagnosis, he lay in bed refusing to take off his pants or socks. It was clear that he had found at least a limited domain in which to exert control!

Jenny was extremely subdued in the weeks following her diagnosis. As much as she had been looking forward to leaving the hospital, she found the homecoming a difficult adjustment. Jenny articulated how different she now felt from the rest of the world, a reality that she had not had to confront while in the hospital. Her mother described Jenny's "dark side," when she would turn inward and seem remote for minutes or hours at a time.

An ambivalent reaction to being at home is not uncommon after the initial hospitalization. The familiarity of home—where on one

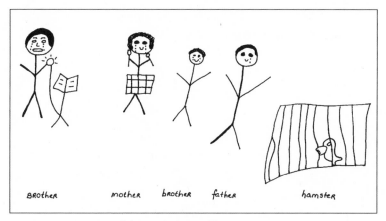

BROTHER   mother   brother   father   hamster

FIGURE I. *Family: I didn't include myself*

level nothing has changed during the hospitalization—is now tinged by the presence of illness. What had previously been protected territory has lost some of that taken-for-granted safety.

Anticipatory grief, the experiential process that reflects the anguish of threatened loss, is precipitated by the diagnosis, and ebbs and flows throughout the course of the illness. While the prognosis for many diseases can now be presented with new optimism, the subjective experience of receiving the diagnosis still connotes death. The following series of drawings illustrates and articulates the inward grief for self and attests to the grief of the family.

A nine-year-old boy portrayed his older brother as a rock singer, his mother cooking, another brother, his father and his pet hamster. When asked what had changed after his diagnosis, he added tears to each person. With regard to the omission of himself he explained: "I didn't include myself, because at the time I was in the hospital and didn't think I'd be back in the picture" (figure I). The little hamster imprisoned in the cage may well be his symbolic self-representation. Thus the boy graphically conveyed his own anticipatory grief.

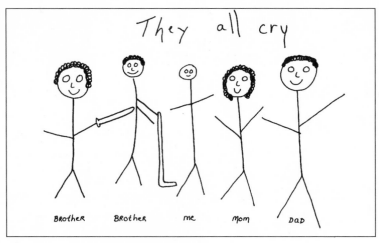

FIGURE 2. *Family: They all cry*

An eight-year-old boy hastily drew stick figures to illustrate the members of his family (figure 2). One brother was playing baseball, another playing hockey, and the patient himself was bald, had no mouth, and was not doing anything. Neither were the parents engaged in any activity. When asked what changed in his family after he became ill, the boy immediately scrawled: "They all cry." This is a striking portrait of anticipatory grief within the family system.[7]

A ten-year-old boy, who had been diagnosed at the age of six, drew an active and engaging family portrait. When asked what had changed after he got sick, he added slashes of rain to the sky. He then crossed out his little brother with the commentary: "My little brother wasn't alive then." His choice of words—"wasn't alive then"—rather than "wasn't born yet" attests to the valence of the life-death dichotomy of the diagnosis. He added tears to his mother and showed his father thinking, "poor kid." He erased himself playing ball and reportrayed himself as he was then—in a wheelchair (figures 3 and 4).

The child's previous experiences with loss bear significantly on his or her reaction to the diagnosis, its meaning and portent. Thus, a

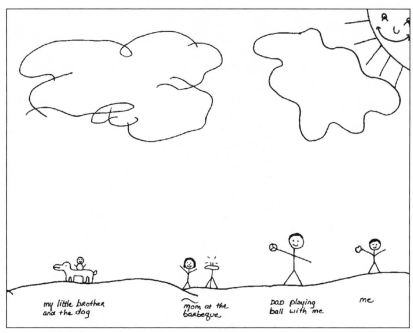

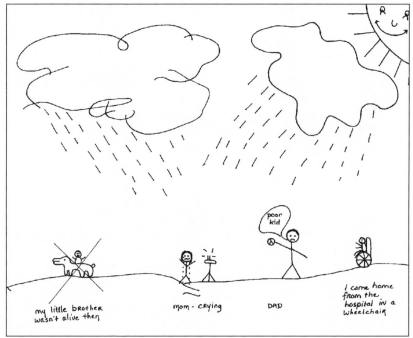

FIGURES 3 *and* 4. *Family: Sun to rain*

child's "loss history," and response to it, are crucial to obtain. The history encompasses loss in its broadest sense; for example, illness and death, trauma, change in relationships (especially parental divorce), geographical moves. Also powerful is the fact that most children have heard about cancer in the media and, like adults, still associate it with death.

Of enormous impact is the child's past acquaintance with the illness he or she now faces. Has the child known someone with the same disease (particularly another child), and if so, what was its trajectory and outcome? The parents and staff must be prepared for such an eventuality.

An eight-year old boy (whose mandala appears as color plate I) lived in a community where he was the third child in six years to be diagnosed with leukemia. He knew the other two children: one had been in continuous remission for over five years and was considered cured; the other was dying. One day, two months after his own diagnosis, the boy "exploded" (his mother's word) out of the house and disappeared for several hours. On his return, he would only tell his parents that he had gone for a walk. However, in a session with the therapist, he was able to elaborate his feelings of "the walk day" through a mandala: "I wanted to be left alone. I was crying [blue]. I felt sad that my friend is so sick —I chose red for blood. I was remembering how we used to play together in the park. I feel sad [yellow] that I have leukemia. I'm still pale but I think that I'm getting better. Of course I'm mad [orange] that kids like us get sick. Why are so many kids getting it? Why are *we* getting it? I thought about how scary it is that my friend might die [purple] and then even more scary that *I* could die from it. I chose black because I think that dying would be like having a blackout. After my walk I felt better, and hopeful that I would be able to play again [green]." As an afterthought, the boy added: "I hope I'll be like the other kid" (color plate III).

Regardless of past experience, the child soon meets others in the hospital or clinic whose appearance alone is initially frightening. Inextricable with these encounters is the growing recognition that he or she is now one of "them." As the child gradually gains familiarity with the medical routine—albeit difficult and painful—some sense of order is restored. With the abatement of the immediate crisis of diagnosis and the entry into the chronic phase, the child's vision turns toward living in the presence of life-threatening illness.

UNDERSTANDING THE ILLNESS

Coping with the trauma of illness can be facilitated by a cognitive understanding of the disease and its treatment. For this reason, the presentation of accurate information in developmentally meaningful terms is crucial. A general guideline is to follow the child's lead: he or she questions facts or implications only when ready, and that readiness must be respected. It is the adult's responsibility to clarify the precise intent of any question and then to proceed with a step-by-step response, thereby granting the child options at each juncture. He or she may choose to continue listening, to ask for clarification, or to terminate the discussion. Offering *less* information with the explicit invitation to ask for *more* affords a safety gauge of control for the child. When these guidelines are not followed, serious miscommunications may ensue. For example, an adult who hears "What is going to happen to me?" and does not clarify the intent of the query may launch into a long statement of plans or elaborate reassurances. The child may respond with irritation: "I only wanted to know what tests I am going to have tomorrow." In such an instance, the adult has grossly overresponded to a question, flooding the child with much more information than was requested or could be absorbed. In contrast, there are times when he or she *is* referring to broader life-and-death issues that must be addressed. The spontaneity and directness of the child's comments and questions can be startling.

On the way home from the clinic, Jonathan asked: "How did I get 'insolved' in the clinic? What's the name of my disease again? Am I all better now? Did I get all better when they 'translated' [transplanted] my sister's bone marrow into me?"

Whenever a four-year-old boy would hear his mother on the telephone discussing medical issues (regardless of whether or not they pertained to him), he would begin to chant: "No clinic, no medicines."

Karen knew the names and dosages of all her medications. During treatment, she would routinely quiz the nurses as to what and how much of each drug they were giving her. While they were occasionally irritated by her "supervision," they could not help but admire her intellectual means of coping with overwhelming anxiety.

The young child's concrete level of reasoning limits or compromises comprehension. Neither the parents nor the caregiver may be aware that the child is operating under misconceptions, unless he or she spontaneously voices the confusion, or even guilt.

A three-year-old boy had initially been satisfied with the explanation: "You need the medicine to get rid of the booboo in your tummy." Months into his treatment, he protested: "There's nothing wrong with my tummy." His mother explained: "You can't see it—it's inside." The child pulled up his shirt to look.

A four-year-old girl was hospitalized because of her low white blood cell count, which made her highly susceptible to infection. Her confused explanation of the hospitalization was: "I can't go home to see my sister. I can't play with her because I would make her sick. I would make my daddy and my mommy and my friends sick too."

A four-year-old boy had undergone surgery in which his bladder was removed and an external bag to collect urine was attached to the skin on his abdomen. The longing for a new bladder so that he could be rid of the bag was the focus of much of his play. Understandably, he confused the terms "bladder" and "tumor," since both had been removed in the surgery. Thus, to the consternation of the adults around him, the child would often say: "I wish I could get a new tumor." During this period, he would arrange operations for Kiss the Squirrel: "To take out his bladder, and then he gets a new tumor—I mean a new bladder!"

When the physician greeted an eleven-year-old girl at her annual checkup, he cheerfully said: "Let's hear what's going on in your head these days!" The child looked startled, paled, and asked: "Are you worried that my head is going to explode?"

Once a misconception is voiced, the parents or caregiver can work with the child to clarify his or her understanding. Explanatory drawings, the repeating back of new information, and highly structured play are all means of consolidating the learning. However, the correction of the immature viewpoint may have to await the child's cognitive capacity to integrate it. Even after mastering the correct reality, he or she often clings to the concrete reasoning as a "private" version of the facts. This is particularly true of the child who has been diagnosed at a young age. The imprint of the early view, even when it is mostly supplanted by more mature comprehension, may intrude in what appears to be irrational fear or guilt. At this later time, the misconceptions, both factual and now with an emotional overlay, can be worked through more effectively. Given the cognitive complexity inherent in understanding the illness and treatment, the conceptual grasp which most children *do* attain is impressive.

Illness as Punishment

Once home from his initial hospitalization, a three-year-old boy was overheard berating his teddy bear: "Teddy Bear, if you don't shape up, I'm going to take you to the children's hospital. They'll give you needles. If you don't behave then, they'll take you to the clinic. The needles hurt. They kill. *Then* if you don't behave, I'll leave you."[8] In a separate incident a few weeks later, the child was punished and sent to his room. Over the intercom, his parents heard his plea: "Please God. I'll be good. Don't send me back to that hospital."

This child's words attest to the powerful perception of illness as a punishment for wrongdoing and of separation as abandonment. The child's concrete thinking does not easily permit the concept of randomness to have any meaning. Thus, when the illness strikes, he or she assumes that such things could only happen to someone who is bad. On the other hand, the child fights that notion, protesting the injustice of a "good kid" being subjected to such hardship. While "treatment" is a word with positive valence, the young child has difficulty in projecting beyond the immediacy of the physical and mental pain engendered. This view of treatment as punishment leads many children to be as compliant as possible in the medical environment, in the hope that good behavior will be rewarded by less pain.

Whenever a four-year-old girl came into the clinic, she would chant beseechingly, "I'm a good girl, I'm a good girl," as if her words could ward off the painful procedures. A nurse commented: "She keeps looking at you as if to say: 'I'm an okay kid. Why are you doing this to me?' And when you agree that she is a good girl, she just looks at you as if you are a monster when you proceed with what has to be done."

A seven-year-old girl engaged a stuffed squirrel in the following interchange:

Child: Do you mind needles? Do you throw up?
Squirrel: [doesn't answer]
Child: I guess he doesn't mind needles—he's not saying anything.
            That means he's a good patient.

Thus, she defined the good patient as someone who does not protest or complain.

Overcompliance can generalize into the child's daily life outside the medical setting. In such instances, the child develops a polarized view of good/bad, right/wrong, and strives desperately to be correct in behavior or performance.

The girl who had articulated her definition of "the good patient" reported: "A lot of people don't like the teacher I'm getting next year. But my teacher says I'll like her because I'm good and we'll get along. I'm a good girl in school so that I won't get yelled at." In September, she reported: "My teacher yells a lot, but not at me because I'm good. Sometimes I get scared that I could say something wrong, or that I don't understand. Other kids raise their hands, but I don't. I'm afraid of being yelled at. I'm scared of being bad and getting in trouble." The child's obsessive terror about being good or bad was further reflected in the stomachaches that she developed before going to school most mornings.

A six-year-old boy's teacher spontaneously observed that he seemed unnecessarily afraid to make any mistakes in his work.

Some children fall into the opposite trap: that is, they act out the terms of a self-fulfilling prophecy. The belief that one must *be* bad to have brought on the illness leads the child to *behave* badly. The negative responses elicited from others confirm the prophecy and further damage the child's sense of self-worth. The illness thus operates at the core of a vicious cycle.

Both overcompliance and acting-out can be seen as manifestations of the child's belief system regarding the illness. Once the child's misconceptions are recognized, the process of moderating the extreme reactions can begin.

Relationship with the Medical Caregivers

The child's relationship with the physicians and nurses develops over time, often from a starting point of undiluted terror to a profound bond of trust and affection. A six-year-old boy stated proudly: "My doctor is my best friend!" Some children may always remain predominantly fearful of the caregivers, never letting down their guard. However, most children are eventually able to integrate the staff's caring with the necessary infliction of pain that treatment involves.

The assignment of a primary physician and nurse provides an anchoring security to the child. The possessiveness of "*my* doctor" or "*my* nurse" singles these individuals out of the many professionals involved. This is especially important in a teaching institution, where the child must adapt to the frequent rotation of trainees and the disruptive cycle of acquaintanceship, attachment, and departure.

THE BODY

Changes and Disfigurement

Physical changes, whether temporary or permanent effects of treatment or the illness, play a major role in the child's experience. Winnicott's concept of personalization, "not only that the psyche is placed in the body, but also that eventually . . . the whole of the body becomes the dwelling place of the self," emphasizes how central the body is to psychic development.[9] Because a child *inhabits* the body so intensely, any disruption in its form or function will have consequences. Drastic changes in appearance raise the question: Am I the same person as before? The child must internalize the concepts of constancy and change, sameness and difference, in order to coordinate the body with the self. Thus, mastering the concept of an altered body image is both a cognitive and an emotional task. It is often assumed that changes in appearance are less traumatic for the child than for the adolescent or adult. Yet, even a young child recognizes their significance, from the cosmetic surface through their profound testimony to the gravity of the illness. They represent the havoc wrought by the disease and may become the target of the child's expressed grief. Scars, a permanent testimony to trauma, may eventually come to symbolize healing, cure, and even heroism to the child.

In her first session with the therapist, a seven-year-old girl asked: "Do you know my doctor? He does operations on me sometimes. Do you want to see a big scar on my stomach?" Without waiting for an answer, she lifted her blouse and explained: "The scar is where they took out my cancer. It used to hurt a lot, but not any more. Even though I think it's ugly, it reminds me that my cancer is gone."

Acceptance of the temporary hair loss secondary to chemotherapy is initially difficult for most children. Reactions of fear and sadness are common. However, over time, matter-of-fact comments about the baldness—even humor—surface.

When an eleven-year-old girl was asked what had been the hardest part of the illness for her, she answered: "losing my hair." As her drawing indicates, the child felt stripped and vulnerable (figure 5).

A three-year-old boy was acutely aware of his baldness. He would stop to look at his reflection

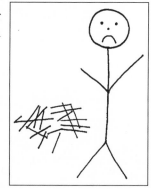

FIGURE 5. *Losing my hair*

in store windows, always with a pained expression, and ask his mother: "Do I look funny?" He was visibly hurt by any comments or stares directed toward him. The issue was excruciatingly highlighted when he asked why his parents didn't have a recent photograph of him in the living room: "Is it because you don't want to have a picture of me bald?" Eventually, the child announced a cheerful compensation for his baldness: it was great not to get shampoo in his eyes!

An eight-year-old girl who had been bald most of her life because of continuous treatment stated: "I like hats. I don't have hair because I take very strong medicine—something in a bottle that makes me very sick. Everyone asks me why I don't have hair. I try to explain it to them, but they don't get it out of their head. Sometimes they laugh at me. It's not very fun. It's not very fair. It makes me mad." She proceeded to draw a picture with the following explanation: "This is Mr. Snail, the groom. He is going to his wedding. He had to brush his hair, so he's late." Her identification with the snail was clear, since, like Mr. Snail, her own head was smooth and shiny and often covered with an interesting hat (figure 6).

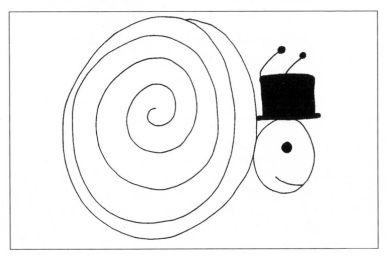

FIGURE 6. *Mr. Snail*

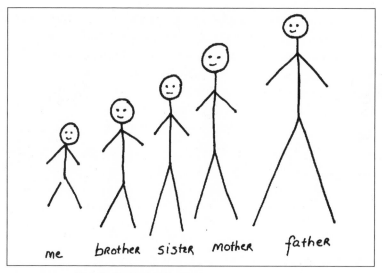

me   bRotheR   sisteR   motheR   fatheR

FIGURE 7. *Family: Losing my leg*

Some children are faced with the loss—or loss of function—of a body part or organ, or with extreme disfigurement. This devastation often occurs as the child is negotiating the immediate impact of the diagnosis and treatment. While mourning the loss of his or her "intactness," the child must simultaneously begin the accommodation to a new body image. For these children, the illness takes on a concrete identity, organized around the core of bodily damage.

A ten-year-old boy had recently had his leg amputated. In response to the question of what had changed most *in the family* since his diagnosis, he answered by scrawling a drawing. He depicted himself as having two legs, although one is severed from the body (figure 7). The boy thus portrayed himself in the process of "letting go" of the leg. In answer to the same question, an eleven-year-old girl who had been paralyzed by a spinal cord tumor stated: "I ended up in a wheelchair" (fig-

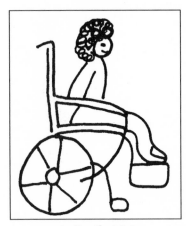

FIGURE 8. *Family: Me in a wheelchair*

ure 8). In both cases, the drastic physical changes in the child's body overwhelmed the salience of any shift in the family system.

After the removal of his bladder, a four-year-old boy referred quite openly to "going home with my bag" (the external bag to collect urine that was attached to the skin on his abdomen). Out of plastic wrap and adhesive, the therapist and the child constructed a bag for Kiss the Squirrel, even marking the same number of stitches as he had. In the months following the operation, most of his drawings were in the shape of a pouch, like a bladder. He drew a lemon filled with predominantly dark, menacing tissue (color plate IV). The pointed end is yellow, reflecting his preoccupation with urination. A second drawing, of a rocking chair, is brighter and less threatening than the lemon (color plate v). The last in the series, a hippopotamus, is a blood-red pouch, somewhat battered by scars (color plate VI).

An eight-year-old girl who had a large tumor in her cheek also had lost her hair and much weight. Prior to the illness, she had been an exceptionally pretty child with almost waist-length hair. In the first few months after her diagnosis, her affect was flat, and she talked very little. Eventually she told the therapist: "I keep looking for myself in the mirror, but I can't find me." In the playroom one day, the child life specialist was taking Polaroid pictures of each child to put into frames that they had designed. This girl studied her photo as the image emerged, making no comment except to ask about her swollen cheek and eye. Over time, one side of her face became increasingly distended. Almost obsessively, she drew a series of puppy dogs, all of whom had "swollen," asymmetrical jowls (figure 9). One of her last drawings was of a little

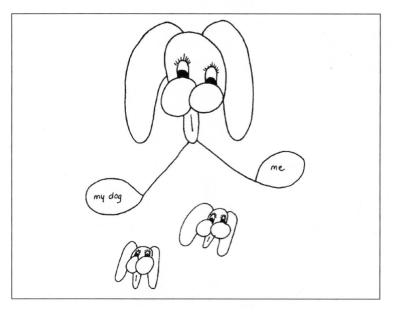

FIGURE 9   *My dog and me*

figure crying. Across the cheeks were two bands. This implicit self-portrait was signed : "From me to everybody" (figure 10).

Reactions to changes in appearance vary from child to child. They wax and wane over time and are influenced to a great extent by the parents' cues. If they can accept the changes—albeit acknowledging sadness and distress—they enable the child to emerge with a core of confidence intact. However, in a family with a narcissistic emphasis on appearance, a pervasive sense of loss or shame complicates the child's adjustment.

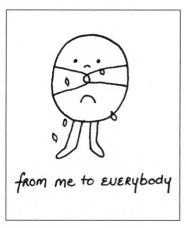

FIGURE 10

Awareness of the Body

He's very in tune with his body. He notices everything.
(mother of a seven-year-old boy)

I hope that my body knows what it's doing. I'm concerned.
(eight-year-old boy)

While the ramifications of illness emanate from the physical to the psychological, the body is its focal site. Thus, not surprisingly, the child develops a heightened awareness of the body, a vigilance that grants at least a limited sense of control. Even a young child possesses "the wisdom of the body," and any observations about changes or symptoms should be heeded. As time goes on, and the child gains distance from the terror of the illness and treatment regimen, the intensity of the watchfulness abates. However, a child who has been through a life-threatening illness never entirely loses that extra awareness. The body—as the embodiment of survival itself—is not taken for granted.

The vigilance only becomes a problem when its intensity develops an obsessive quality. In such cases, the parents may describe their child as a "hypochondriac." The child has learned that illness is a guarantee of the parents' immediate attention, and the reporting of symptoms continues as a means to this end. At least initially the child achieves his or her goal, because parents panic and caregivers worry at the thought of "missing" something. Thus, the differential diagnosis of hypochondriasis in a child with a history of serious illness can be difficult. However, ruminative worry about the body often masks unresolved fears that have no other avenue of expression; or, the child is simply continuing to function "in sickness" because he or she has not yet negotiated the way back to living in health.

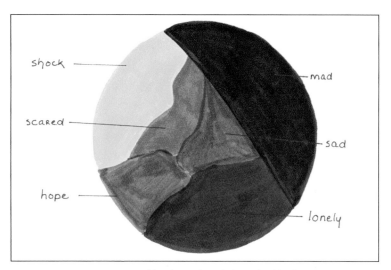

COLOR PLATE I. *How I felt when I heard that I had leukemia*

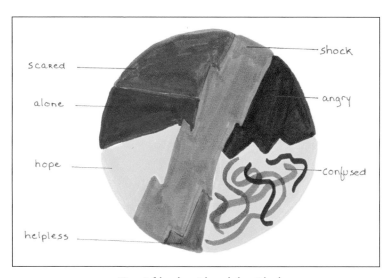

COLOR PLATE II. *How I felt when I heard that I had cancer*

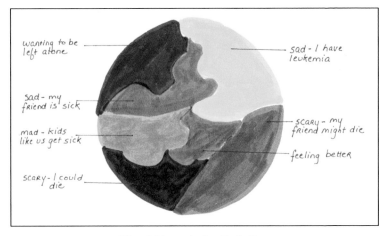

wanting to be
left alone

sad - my
friend is sick

mad - kids
like us get sick

scary - I could
die

sad - I have
leukemia

scary - my
friend might die

feeling better

COLOR PLATE III. *How I felt on the "walk-day"*

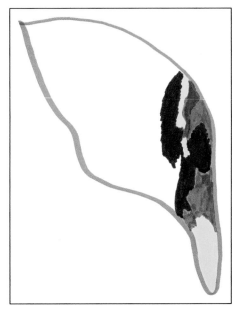

COLOR PLATE IV. *Lemon*

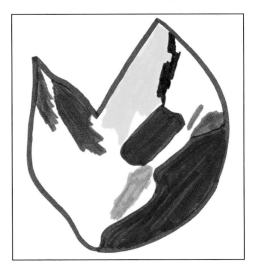

COLOR PLATE V. *Rocking chair*

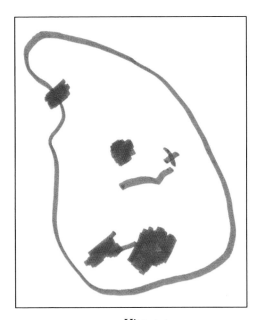

COLOR PLATE VI. *Hippopotamus*

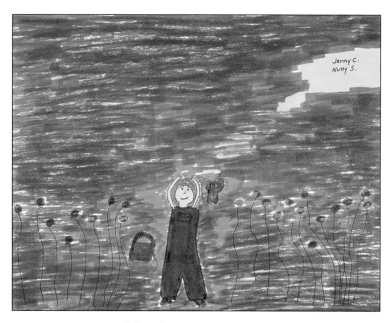

COLOR PLATE VII. *Relaxation scene*

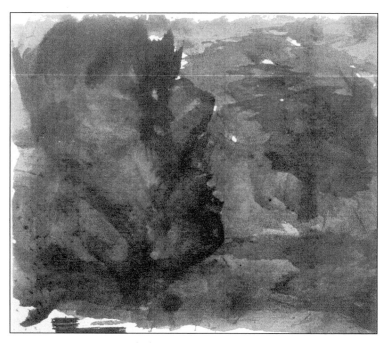

COLOR PLATE VIII. *Black*

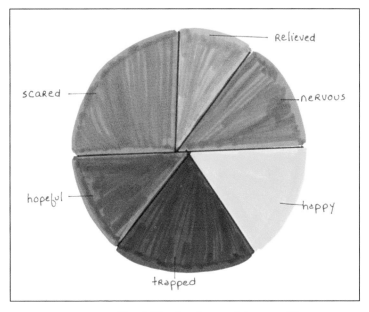

COLOR PLATE IX. *How I felt when I entered the room (K)*

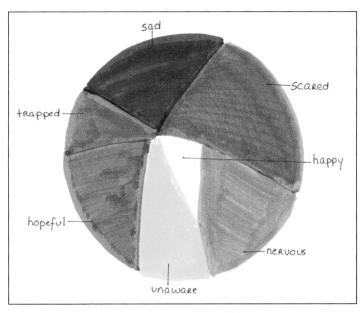

COLOR PLATE X. *How I felt when I entered the room (S)*

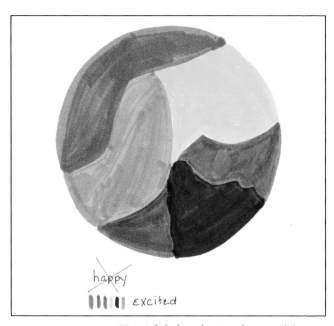

COLOR PLATE XI. *How I feel about leaving the room (K)*

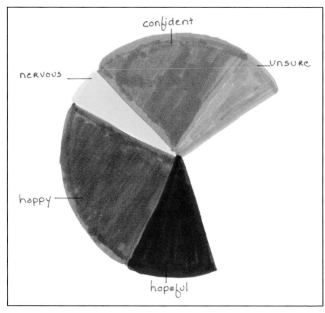

COLOR PLATE XII. *How I feel about leaving the room (S)*

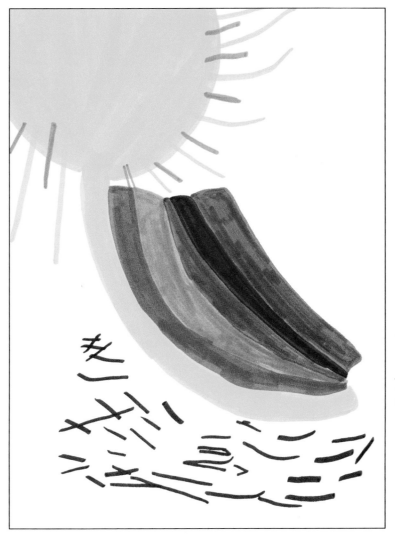

COLOR PLATE XIII. *Rainbow*

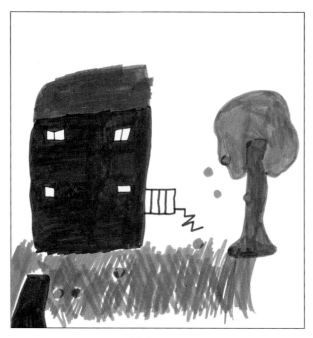

COLOR PLATE XIV. *My house*

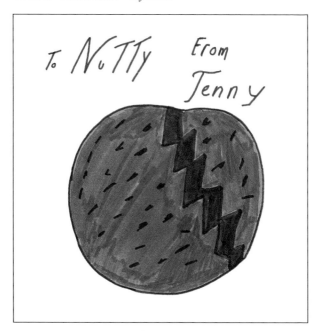

COLOR PLATE XV. *Walnut*

The mind-body connection is firmly entrenched in a child who has been seriously ill. Psychosomatic symptoms—either inextricably tied to the illness itself or related to more general stress—may emerge as a route of expression. In the following examples, the interweaving is evident.

In the months after completing treatment, a five-year-old boy gained a huge amount of weight. He explained spontaneously: "I'm building a strong wall so that the bad leukemia cells can't hurt me again."

Karen complained that her body hurt whenever anyone in the family got angry at her. In discussion with the therapist, she was eventually able to define the pain more precisely as feeling tense.

Touch

Poly Polar Bear loves to be loved, cuddled and held close. This makes him feel happy and makes his hardships seem a little easier.[10]

Touch is comforting for the seriously ill child as an antidote to pain and anxiety and as reassurance of the presence of others. For the child whose body has been probed and invaded, the relief of soothing contact is enormous. Furthermore, touch reassures the child that he or she is neither ugly nor "untouchable" and counteracts feelings of shame or fear of the revulsion by others. The very nature of touch is intensely personal, and both psychological and cultural factors affect its expression. Thus, the capacity of an individual (a family member or caregiver) for physical demonstrativeness must be respected. Parents who have not been comfortable with touch in the past need guidance about its importance for their child in the current circumstances. Even parents who are demonstrative may shy away, intimidated by the medical equipment, or simply overwhelmed by the child's fragility. The therapist can model the use of touch for both parents and the professional team, emphasizing its effectiveness as a therapeutic tool, as well as a "way of being" in relationship to the child.

A hospitalized eight-year-old girl would become extremely anxious at bedtime. She chattered incessantly, fighting to stay awake. One evening, the therapist stroked the child's leg through the blanket while they talked. Within minutes, she had fallen asleep. The next day, the girl exclaimed: "You found a new way to make me sleep!" The therapist demonstrated the "technique" to her parents, who were then able to soothe her.

A ten-year-old boy would cry and turn away in distress whenever a nurse came to check the flow of his medication through the tubing. The therapist suggested that the nurse always put her arm around him for a few seconds before approaching the equipment. Within a few instances of this intervention, the child's agitation ceased entirely.

The use of touch by the therapist raises issues particular to that role. While the boundary for touching a patient who is a seriously ill child is more flexible than in traditional psychotherapy, caution must nonetheless be exercised and the rationale for its use evaluated. Spontaneous hugs of greeting, sitting near the child, adopting an approachable posture, touching or holding the child—all these are part of the intimacy of the therapeutic relationship. Furthermore, the therapist who accompanies the child for any sort of procedure will invariably be involved in physical contact. It is crucial, however, that the therapist not be emotionally seductive to the child through touch. This is especially so if there is any history of sexual inappropriateness or abuse in the family. When used carefully and selectively by the therapist, touch can be a powerful affirmation of connectedness during a time of threatened loss.

MEDICAL PROCEDURES

Sometimes I feel like a test tube, just having different medicines being pushed into me. (Karen)

The child must develop strategies to confront time and time again the painful procedures of investigation and treatment. As a seven-year-old girl explained: "I used to watch the IV fill up to get used to it. Now I'm used to it." Then, as an afterthought she added: "You never *really* get used to it all, but you have to." The theme of habituation is one that children verbalize often, with a matter-of-factness that offsets any passive resignation. In fact, "getting used to something" affords the child a certain degree of control, albeit within the limits of having no choice but to submit. Natalie Kusz addresses this theme in her memoir: "Surgery, I thought, was a necessary evil, and I had no choice but to walk through it in the best way I had, holding close to those who went with me." She also describes the behavior of a three-year-old child with leukemia whom she had known on the ward: "His mother was usually the one to draw him away from our games when it was time for treatments, and although he knew what was coming, he never ran from it; when he asked his mother, 'Do I have to?' it was not a protest, but a question, and when she replied that yes, this was necessary, he would accept her hand and leave the playroom on his feet."[11]

Certainly the child's acceptance of the treatment regimen is based upon a recognition, implicit or explicit, of the gravity of the illness.

Jenny informed the therapist: "Chemo causes hair loss and vomiting, and I hate that, but I would die without the chemo. I'd rather lose my hair than die. This is the medicine that keeps me alive."

Although "getting used to" serves the child well for a certain period, it may falter as time goes on. From the initial period of terror, through the gradual adaptation, the child may, in a different phase, once again experience extreme difficulty in tolerating the regimen.

Drawings

In the following series of drawings, children convey their terror and powerlessness in facing the onslaught of treatment. They portray an encapsulated reality, at times shocking in its starkness. Many of these pictures were drawn to represent the child's "scariest" experience.

A four-year-old boy spontaneously drew "a slingshot, stone, cup and blood" in the hour prior to his chemotherapy infusion at the clinic (figure 11). The drawing virtually crackles with agitation and chaos. While he could not explain his choice of objects, the slingshot— a weapon of assault causing injury— speaks for itself. In another session, he addressed the challenges of treatment in more contained fashion. With great concentration, he filled out a clinic appointment card, "translating" what he had written as: "IV rules: Do not kick. Do not scream. Do not pull your hand away" (figure 12).

In the next drawing (figure 13), a six-year-old boy explained the bone marrow aspiration: "It's a big needle.

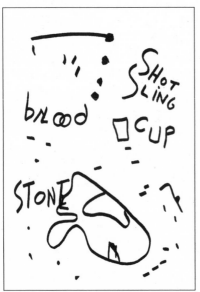

FIGURE 11. *Slingshot, stone, cup, and blood*

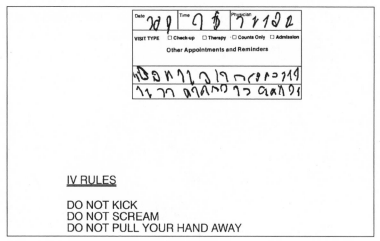

FIGURE 12. *IV rules*

They stick it in your back and wind it. If you had one, you'd be screaming! I try to run away. I hate to get shots in my back—that's where all my bones is." He did not represent himself in the picture. This omission, a form of dissociation, allows the child a measure of distance from the horror that he or she has endured. As a defense against being overwhelmed, it is common in drawings of painful

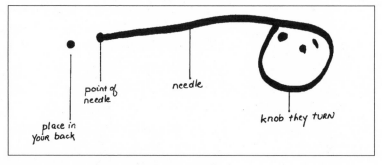

FIGURE 13. *Bone marrow aspiration needle*

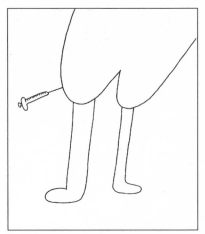

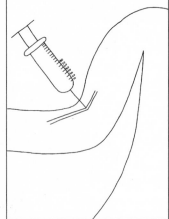

FIGURE 14. *Needle in the butt*   FIGURE 15. *Needle in the arm*

procedures. After completing the bone marrow aspiration needle, the child asked the therapist: "Does it hurt when a tooth falls out?" Such is the dramatic juxtaposition of the ordinary and the extraordinary in the life of a six-year-old with a life-threatening illness!

Figures 14 and 15 illustrate the invasiveness of needles.[12] These drawings were done in a group setting and sparked a lively debate as to whether needles in the "butt" are worse than needles in the arm. Both pictures demonstrate a type of partial dissociation: the full body of the child is omitted; only parts are suggested. The ten-year-old boy who drew the needle "in the butt" had actually had a leg amputated. Although the leg is not severed as in another of his pictures (figure 7), he does depict it as being "less present" by virtue of its being thinner and shorter than the existent leg. In the eleven-year-old girl's drawing of the needle in the arm, the precise markings on the syringe attest to the extreme vigilance that many children maintain over their treatment.

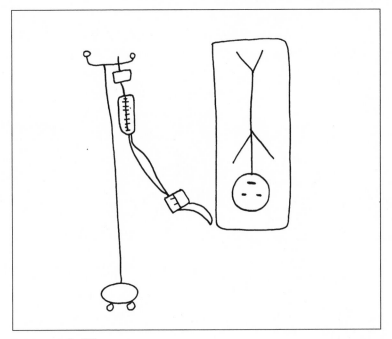

FIGURE 16. *IV*

The next two images are menacing and horrific. In figure 16, drawn by an eight-year-old boy, the intravenous tubing does not even touch the skeletal child, who looks as if he is entombed in a coffin. This disconnection from the medical equipment may represent another form of protective dissociation, or the child may be communicating a terrified skepticism as to the treatment's value for himself. In figure 17, an eleven-year-old girl recounted: "Once you're sick, you don't even feel like a human being any more. They just do things to you as if you're some kind of robot." The masked physician's hands, grossly distorted in size and shape, touch neither of the two syringes in the humanoid body of the patient.

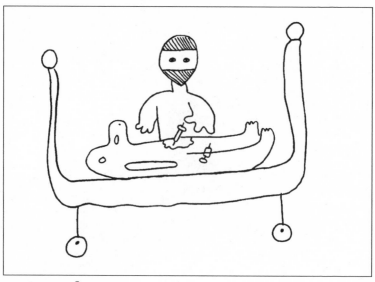

FIGURE 17. *Surgery*

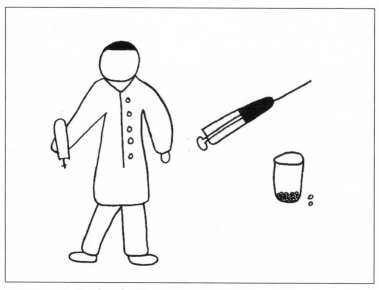

FIGURE 18. *Faceless physician*

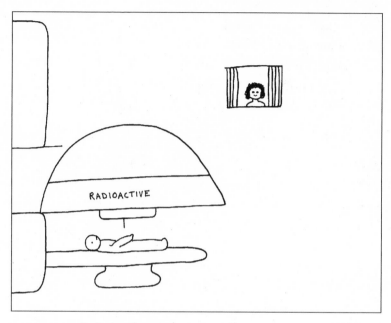

FIGURE 19. *Radiation therapy*

The drawings often depict caregivers anonymously or omit them entirely. In an image by an eleven-year-old boy (figure 18), the physician is faceless. The child's explanation was typical: "I really like my doctors and nurses, and I know they hate to hurt me. So I don't want to put them in my pictures of these awful things." Thus, the lack of identification, or outright omission of the caregiver, may be the child's means of protecting the relationship from his or her anguish and anger.

Radiation therapy and imaging techniques are portrayed less frequently than the invasive procedures. Yet, figure 19 illustrates the vulnerability of an eleven-year-old girl lying under a machine getting radiation therapy. She is alone, but for the intercom contact with the technician behind the window. The child confessed: "I was always afraid that the machine would fall on me." This fear is prevalent, although often unspoken, among children overwhelmed by the sheer enormity of the apparatus and its various noises when in operation. Furthermore, the child labeled the machine (and thus herself?) "radioactive."

Medical Play

The children's drawings certainly attest to the unrelenting assault of life-threatening illness. In play with stuffed animals, using the medical equipment itself, a different quality of expression emerges. The children "treat," converse with, question, and berate the animals, all the while commiserating with one another's plight. Humor and enjoyment infuse the interactive play. In the following excerpt from a psychotherapy session, the utter seriousness of the message is playfully conveyed:

The therapist commented: "Nutty the Squirrel hates having leukemia." Jenny retorted immediately: "I'm with you Nutty!" She then delivered the following lecture to him: "You don't understand what we're doing to you. You need information. Leukemia is a disease for which you need medicines. If you don't take medicine, you could get into serious trouble. You could die and not live any more and you wouldn't be able to eat walnuts. So you have to cooperate if you want to be able to eat walnuts." She then picked up Snoopy, who was wearing a doctor's gown and mask, and introduced him to Nutty: "Snoopy is a vet. He takes care of rabies, colds, pneumonia, and a couple of leukemia patients. He's no ordinary doctor!"

The children's engagement in the medical play with the animals is intensely concentrated.

A five-year-old girl involved several animals in a hospital scenario, mimicking terms that she had heard in her own experience. "Curious

George needs blood. He has low counts and 'aminonia' [pneumonia]. Tommy Lobster needs blood too. I have to check their ears. Wait a minute—I don't think lobsters have ears—I think they're like snakes!" In the next session, the play continued. "Curious George has measles and chicken pox and mumps. He's throwing up from his medicines. He needs a lot of liquids and only half a banana a day. One vitamin at night, and two when he wakes up. Snoopy can take care of him at night, but he has to remember to wear a mask." The girl's departing words at the end of the session were: "I'm changing the orders for Curious George—vitamins three times a day."

The process of identification with the animal becomes the crucial pivot of the communication.

Karen was preparing to start an IV on Poly Polar Bear. "Even if it's only pretend, I hate to put it in him even for a minute," she sighed.

A four-year-old boy informed the therapist: "My teddy bear doesn't cry when he gets needles." The therapist responded: "I know you cry when you get them. I wonder why your teddy bear doesn't." The child replied matter-of-factly: "Because I have a lot of leukemia and he has only a little."

A seven-year-old girl was treating Curious George, who was thrashing around and resisting her. She became very angry: "I had it much worse than you! I had it when I was only two years old, and you're four—so stop fussing!"

When offered the option of using either animals or dolls in medical play, the child tends to select animals. It is possible that they pose a less direct threat than a representation of a human. In turn, the child may feel freer to exert his or her authority over animals, enhancing a sense of control. Some children are attracted to the cuddliness of a stuffed animal. Nonetheless, dolls do elicit many of the same concerns.

Over the course of several sessions, Jonathan played repetitive versions of the same scenario with dollhouse figures and an ambulance. In one session, he had the baby get sick, followed by the girl and boy. Then the parents got hurt. The whole family went to the hospital by ambulance. The baby kept asking: "What's happening?" "Don't be scared, baby," would always be the answer. Everyone got X-rays at the hospital, and one by one, they all were proclaimed "better." What was particularly interesting in Jonathan's stories was that he always had everybody be ill, as if to counteract the lonely reality of being the only patient in his own family.

Relaxation and Hypnosis Techniques

Relaxation and hypnosis techniques can be extremely effective in symptom control; for example, to reduce discomfort related to procedures and nausea, as well as for insomnia and general anxiety. Even when the techniques do not *objectively* ameliorate a symptom, most children *subjectively* report an increased sense of self-control in using the imagery. Children are imaginative in constructing images that distract or remove the focus from what they are undergoing. The child may evoke a scene (possibly integrating the therapeutic stuffed animal), visualize familiar characters from television or books, or simply use a standard relaxation image. Whatever the choice, having the child draw a picture of the scene heightens its realism and detail. Once the therapist has recorded the relaxation tape, his or her voice reinforces a certain security and continuity for the child.

An eight-year-old girl who had been a swimming champion before her illness chose the following image as her focus: "I'm doing laps in the pool, and my mother is swimming beside me." She thus combined pleasurable activity, achievement, and health with the security of her mother's presence.

Karen incorporated Poly Polar Bear, her most comforting companion, into an image of "flying on a cottony-white Poly Polar Bear cloud" far from the world of needles and pain.

Jenny's relaxation scene, an antidote to nausea associated with chemotherapy, was to be lying in a field of flowers on a warm, sunny day with Nutty the Squirrel. She would be barefoot, wearing overalls. They would have a picnic basket filled with both their favorite foods: nut soup, chicken rice soup, sandwiches, lasagna, cookies, candy, ice cream, apples, and milk. The importance of her companionship with Nutty, as well as the link with the therapist, was indicated by the signature on the picture. She included the initials of her own and the therapist's last name: "Jenny C. and Nutty S." (color plate VII).

HOSPITALIZATION

When Ricky was asked who would be visiting him in the hospital, he listed many family members, but did not include his mother. When the therapist commented on the omission, he retorted indignantly: "My mother doesn't visit me—she *stays* with me!" [13]

On her return home after a long hospitalization, a four-year-old girl greeted her parents and sister: "I lost you and now you're back!"

These exclamations show how profound the separation engendered by hospitalization can feel to a child. Whether or not articulated, the intensity of the reaction derives from the threatening circumstances of the illness. The following drawings graphically convey the vulnerability and aloneness experienced by the hospitalized child.

During each of his hospitalizations, a three-year-old boy followed the identical ritual in his drawings: he would dash some paint on a sheet of paper and then wash over everything with black (color plate VIII). At

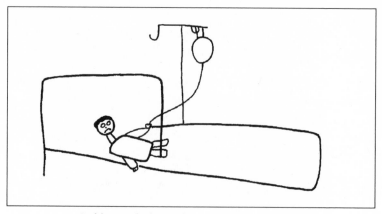

FIGURE 20. *Sad boy in the hospital*

one point, he had eleven such drawings taped on the wall next to his bed! The child's demeanor in the hospital was remarkably outgoing and cheerful; obviously his sense of threat and foreboding was channelled into these pictures. In figure 20, a child lies at an angle, part way out of the bed. His position, like the bed itself, looks precarious. The seven-year-old girl who had drawn the picture said: "It's a sad boy. He wishes he could get out of the hospital." In figure 21, by a ten-year-old girl, the child lies in her bed in stark isolation, accompanied only by an ominous-looking television set.[14] Ricky drew figure 22 on the day before he entered the isolation room. He had just informed the therapist that people would have to wear mask, gown, and gloves when they came in to see him. He took a crayon and carefully delineated a spiral, announcing that it was "a spaceship." Thus he conveyed his understanding of the "high-tech" encapsulation he was about to enter.

Donald Winnicott emphasized the "capacity to be alone" as a crucial sign of maturity in emotional development. The necessary condition for that capacity is the mother's involved presence in the child's early life. Therein lies the paradox. The capacity to be alone is "the experience of being alone while someone else is present.... In

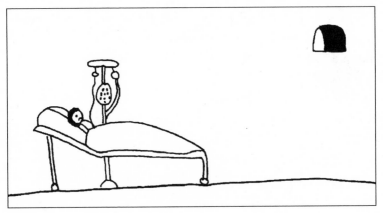

FIGURE 21. *Alone in the hospital*

the course of time, the individual becomes able to forego the *actual* presence of the mother or mother-figure. This has been referred to in such terms as the establishment of an 'internal environment.'"[15]

In light of Winnicott's theory, one realizes how extraordinary are the demands placed on the hospitalized child's psychic functioning. The hospital is intrinsically a strange and frightening environment, whatever the nature and duration of the admission. A child who may not yet possess the cognitive and emotional structures to cope with "aloneness" is thrust into a world where being alone is a sine qua non of the experience. The trauma of hospitalization is somewhat mitigated for a child who can rely on the internal representation of another person's presence. However, for the child who lacks such maturation, either for developmental or

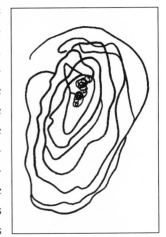

FIGURE 22. *Spaceship*

clinical reasons, the risk for depression and feelings of abandonment is heightened. Prolonged confinement in isolation, when the child's outward mobility as well as incoming visitors are restricted, dramatically exacerbates the stress.

The recognition of the developmental process in a child's ability to be alone has opened the way for parents' presence in the hospital. While most hospitals now allow or even encourage parents to be with the child as much as possible, circumstances arise when a parent simply cannot stay over long periods. Reasons include job demands, siblings at home, distance from the treatment center, and exhaustion. Often, it is the mother who stays and the father who can only come in periodically, and so the child's loneliness is often directed toward missing the father.

A four-year-old boy had been in a room on a bone marrow transplant ward for several months. Since his family lived far from the hospital, his father was only able to visit on weekends. In the week before he was scheduled to leave the room, the child drew a four-part picture with the therapist (figure 23). First he showed "my house where my teddy bear and I will go when we leave the room." The second part continued: "The barn for my teddy bear and me." The therapist then asked the child to draw a picture of what he missed most while in the room. He said instantly and enthusiastically, "My Dad!!!" and drew him. But the mention of his father suddenly catapulted the child into the vulnerability of missing him. His affect changed markedly to sadness and anxiety, and he quickly scrawled a fourth picture that he referred to despondently as "a crooked old house." He then asked to end the session.

Ricky longed to go home from the hospital. He lived in a city distant from the treatment center. The therapist's reference to Poly Polar Bear (whom Ricky had left at home for this admission) led to the disclosure about missing his father.

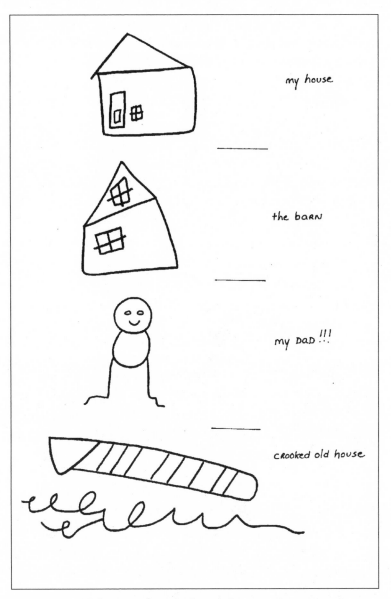

my house

the barn

my dad !!!

crooked old house

FIGURE 23. *My house, my barn, and my dad*

Therapist: Are the headaches better these days?

Ricky: Uh-huh. They're going to be even better when I get more sleep at home. Because that neighborhood has a lot of peace and quiet.

Therapist: And you told me that the doctor said that magic word about . . . what was his magic word that you told me?

Ricky: Going home.

Therapist: Going home. That's a very magic word for you, isn't it?

Ricky: Yah.

Therapist: I bet that Poly Polar Bear is missing you.

Ricky: I bet he's crying.

Therapist: I bet he's crying too. Just like you cry because you miss him.

Ricky: And I miss Daddy.

When parents cannot or do not come in often or for long periods, the child's reactions may encompass longing, withdrawal, and anger.

A four-year-old child would sit at the elevator all day, talking about his parents to whomever passed. When his parents would finally step off the elevator each evening, he would ignore them.

This particularly dramatic example illustrates how interminable a day in the hospital can feel for a child, and how "unreal" it is when the wished-for parents actually arrive. It is as if the child, having coped all day in their absence, cannot suddenly assimilate their presence. Or, perhaps, the child does not let down his or her guard, knowing that the parents will soon leave again. The child's refusal to acknowledge the parents may also be understood as retaliation for the perceived abandonment.

While the hospitalized child misses his or her siblings, the intensity is less. The longing for parents is associated with the fear of being unprotected. This feeling may emerge with regard to older siblings who play something of a parental role, at times even substituting for the parents in the hospital. However, some children report candidly that as much as they miss their brothers and sisters, it is difficult to see and hear of their active lives.

A young child's fear in the hospital may be so profound that even the parents' leaving the room for short periods can be hard to tolerate.

Ricky knew that the isolation room was technically referred to as "protective care." His mother had stayed with him day and night throughout the hospitalization and was totally exhausted.

Ricky: Sometimes children's mommies don't stay with them when they're in protective care.

Therapist: Did your mommy stay with you when you were in protective care?

Ricky: Yah, but she had to go back upstairs because my nurses were very mean then, very mean and nasty.

Therapist: They were mean and nasty because they thought your mother should rest upstairs? [in a room for parents]

Ricky: [nodding]

Therapist: And you didn't like being alone, did you?

Ricky: No. That's why I wasn't very protected.

Obviously, Ricky's definition of "protective care" revolved around the absolute and constant presence of his mother. On a subsequent hospitalization, he reported that he had not been too scared "because Mommy and Daddy were keeping an eye on me all morning and all night. See?" (He pointed to the two chairs in the room.) The discussion continued:

Therapist: Are you feeling better than when you came into the hospital?

Ricky: NO.

Therapist: Worse?

Ricky: Uh-huh.

Therapist: What feels worse?
Ricky: [stating the obvious] That it's not at home.
Therapist: I remember how you said that sometimes you woke up in the middle of the night and that you were lonely and that made you cry.
Ricky: Oh, that made me cry *all the time.*

At certain times, the hospital represents safety to the child, and his or her relief at being surrounded by the caregiving staff is palpable. For the child who has been hospitalized frequently, or for a prolonged period, the hospital becomes a second home. In fact, some children may develop such a sense of security that they need a great deal of preparation for their leave-taking. This is especially true for the child whose family situation is difficult or chaotic and for whom the hospital provides stability. In addition, some children find protection "on the inside" from the insensitivities of the outside world of the healthy. Natalie Kusz remembers:

"A stay in the hospital was for me not confinement, but refuge. In this place, children did not ridicule shaven heads, did not tear at my bandages, did not care to know how many names I would swallow before I started to cry."[16]

Whatever the nature of the child's hospitalization experience, an element of ambivalence is invariably present. While the child may dread the need for the hospital, he or she also depends on its being close at hand "just in case."

Jenny reacted to the family's planned move with panic: "How will we find our way to the hospital from the new house?" Similarly, an eight-year-old child worried about how far the family would be from the hospital during their vacation.

The frequency and duration of hospitalizations varies from child to child, depending on the nature and course of the illness. A "very hospitalized child" creates a life encapsulated within the walls of the hospital, whereas one whose illness is managed predominantly on an out-patient basis leads a more balanced life in the wider world.

BONE MARROW TRANSPLANTATION

Bone marrow transplantation, highly experimental only a decade ago, is now used as a treatment of choice for some childhood illnesses, as well as for tumors that don't respond to initial therapy, or for those that recur.[17] The transplant procedure itself involves high doses of chemotherapy, with or without total body irradiation, followed by infusion of bone marrow. Confinement to a protected room for a period of weeks or months while awaiting the marrow to "take" is required. This relative isolation, whereby the child cannot leave the room, is the hallmark of the experience and intensifies both its drama and its stress. Because bone marrow transplantation is not yet done in every hospital, the child may have to go to another institution for the procedure, often in a distant city. The geographical dislocation only exacerbates the separation issues already being faced, since the child and family are deprived of the support of extended family, friends, and the familiar hospital staff.

A transplant may be autologous, in which the child's own marrow is removed, treated, and returned; or allogeneic, using marrow that is donated, most frequently by a sibling who is a "match." The child perceives the donor sibling as his or her potential savior, and the children often become closer as a result.

The consent process for bone marrow transplantation is fraught with trepidation and hope, both raised to a pitch of great intensity.

Preparation for the procedure must take into account medical, psychological, and logistical concerns.

Jenny wrote a list of questions for the professional team a few weeks before her bone marrow transplantation. She already had had lengthy discussions with her physician about the actual procedures involved. Jenny posed each question as if she were conducting an interview, recording the answers as she received them. The list proceeded as follows: "Can I have things on the wall? [Yes.] How much storage space? [Almost none.] Can I bring in my own quilt and curtains? [Quilt, yes; curtains, no.] How long does the cleaning of my stuff take? [Depends.] Am I going to be in a regular room first? [Don't know yet.] Can I bring an X-mas tree? [Yes, an artificial one.] Can we bring food in? Do I have a window? Can I put on makeup? [No.] Can I wear clothes? [Yes.] Am I being on prenizone [sic]? [No.] Can I bring clarinet? [Yes.] Do I have to have counts every day? [Yes.]" At the end of the questions, she carefully folded the list into her pocket and said she was ready.

The older child may ask to read or hear the informed consent document itself. The form is unsparing in its specificity of risks, including death. Sterility, a likely although not absolute consequence of the procedure, is a long-term effect whose impact is felt by the child in projecting into his or her potential future.

Jenny listened to her physician read the lengthy consent form, interrupting frequently to question or to complain about "too many big words."

Jenny: What does "sterility" mean?
Physician: It means you can't have babies when you grow up.
Jenny: I can't have children? THAT STINKS.... Well, I'll adopt some.[18]

The word "lethal" had been used several times in the document before Jenny asked its meaning. She showed no visible reaction when her physician responded: "It means that you could die of it." After hearing the entire consent form, Jenny proudly signed "on my own line," distinct from the space for a parent or guardian.

The entry into the protected environment, whether it be an elaborate laminar flow room or a germ-free hospital room, is often experienced as a dramatic point of no return. Heightening the anxiety is the reality of the isolation and entrapment. The period of chemotherapy and radiation is harsh for the child to undergo and for the parents to witness. Somewhat paradoxically, the actual infusion of the marrow—the transplant itself—is anticlimactic. The child and family often comment on how innocuous the procedure seems in light of its life-saving potential.

The posttransplant period of waiting for the marrow to take is highly stressful. For the child, family, and staff, the pendulum swings between fear and hope. It is during this time that the child's psychological resources are most challenged. Boredom, frustration, depression, and anger are all common reactions, and the extreme physical confinement affords few outlets. The child wages battles (often around compliance with the medication regimen) with both staff and parents. Careful negotiation is required to allow the child some sense of control in what is, in fact, an overwhelmingly powerless position.

When the procedure is completed, there must be preparation for the child's discharge from the protected environment. While he or she longs to escape from the room, there is often great trepidation about safety on the outside. Exuberance tempered by fear is a frequent reaction to the leave-taking.

On the day of his discharge, a four-year-old boy had packed all his possessions hours before his parents' arrival. "I'm ready to get out of here!" he exclaimed. Later that morning, when it was time to leave the room, he ventured out a few feet into the hall, then turned around and darted back in. He informed everyone that it would be "okay" with him if he didn't go home until the next day. Eventually his parents had to carry him out of the room, accompanied by his protests. When the boy appeared in the clinic the next day, he complained of pain in his legs. What emerged was that on his arrival home, he had run around from room to room for hours, reveling in his newly found freedom of space.

Another factor in leaving the room is the loss of relationships with the staff. A unique intensity and intimacy develops between the child and caregivers within the confinement of the room. Thus, sadness and anticipatory "missing" are an expectable part of the child's reaction to discharge.

The mandalas of two twelve-year-old girls, K and S, convey many facets of the experience of bone marrow transplantation.[19] A few weeks into the procedure, the girls were asked to reflect on how they had felt when they first *entered* the room. The list of feelings that they were given included: scared, mad, alone, sad, trapped, hopeful.

K added relieved, nervous, and happy to the selection of feelings, and rejected mad, alone, and sad. In K's mandala (color plate IX), her need to impose order and control on her intense feelings is evident in the strictly demarcated lines, drawn with a ruler. Just days before entering the room, she had said to the staff: "Remember—I call all the shots!" K gave "scared" both priority and power, by drawing it first, in red. She followed "scared" with "relieved," as if immediately to defuse its intensity. She added "nervous" without explanation and then counterbalanced it with "happy." "Trapped" elicited her most emphatic explanation (incorporating a sense of guilt and punishment), followed by the ending note of "hopeful." K offered the following commentary upon completion of the mandala:

Yes, I was *scared. Relieved* that I was going to get this over with. *Happy* that I was going to have this done and wouldn't have to come back to the hospital ... well, I'd have to come back, but I'd hopefully not have to come back. *Trapped*—yes! Locked up like a prisoner. Being punished for a crime you didn't commit. Being put away. Feeling like you did something wrong, but you didn't.

In S's mandala about entering the room (color plate x), she added the feelings of nervous and unaware and rejected mad and alone. She drew "sad" first, flanked by "scared" (the largest area) and "trapped." Although "hopeful" occupies significant space in the mandala, she did not comment on it. "Unaware" and "nervous" elaborate the sense of uncertainty. "Happy" was added as an almost superstitious afterthought to the remaining area of the circle. S stated:

Blue is a good color for *sad,* because when you're blue, you're sad. *Trapped*—that's it—you really feel that way. *Unaware*—I knew about transplant, but I didn't know exactly what it would be like. I was *nervous* about it. *Scared* ... yes I was scared ... scared that something might happen. The middle is *happy,* because inside I felt a little happy that I could have the transplant.

The girls' reactions to *leaving* the room and going home were elicited in a mandala the morning of their discharge. The list of feelings included: happy, relieved, nervous, confident, hopeful. K stated about her mandala, with its restored fluidity of feelings (color plate xi):

I feel happy, just happy.... No, not happy. Excited. Just excited. All the bright colors. Like a rainbow swirling around.

S omitted "relieved" and added "unsure" to her list (color plate xii). She began with "confident," proceeded through "nervous" and "unsure," and ended with "happy" and "hopeful." In allocating a significant proportion of the circle to "happy," she stated:

I am just happy to go home and see my dog.

She thus focused her positive feeling on the anticipated reunion, rather than on the successful outcome of the transplantation itself. S could not ascribe a feeling to the white space, which lurks somewhat threateningly in its emptiness.

Both girls highlighted feeling "trapped" when they embarked on the transplant procedure. Beyond the confinement of the room itself, "trapped" compellingly symbolizes the extreme circumstances in which the child is caught. The girls seemed to distinguish between the anxious uncertainty of "nervous" and the more profound "scared." "Hope" was represented in all the mandalas. The omission of "anger" and "alone" is significant. The child undergoing such high-risk treatment may simply be too frightened to express anger. Furthermore, the vulnerability and extreme dependence on others for both physical and psychological survival makes its expression a threatening proposition. Several weeks out of the transplant room, K suggested that horror films be purchased for bone marrow transplant patients, "so that they can scream and get all their anger out." The denial of "alone" may be necessary in order for the child to cope with the already profound sense of isolation.

K's mandalas moved from a state of rigid constriction to a depiction of life in flowing motion once again. She had undergone transplantation as the first choice of treatment for her disease and embarked on it with fear coupled with great hope. The doubtful, less assured quality of S's mandalas reflected the fact that she had had multiple relapses of her disease, and the procedure for her was a treatment of last resort. The girls' mandalas illustrate how the emotional reverberations of the same procedure can differ depending on the prognosis for its outcome.

The readjustment to the wider world after transplantation can be difficult, in that the child may continue to exhibit quite fearful and dependent behavior, and family relationships and roles may undergo reorganization. If the parents are given realistic expectations for the days, weeks, and months ahead, they can buffer this transition period both for the child and for the family as a whole.

ELECTIVE CESSATION OF TREATMENT

The term *elective cessation* refers to the discontinuation of all forms of therapy at a time when the disease is judged to have been adequately treated.[20] While the regimen may have included surgery and radiation therapy, in terms of elective cessation, chemotherapy is most often the issue. As children survive for longer periods of time, this new and critical milestone has emerged.

Parents often express extreme ambivalence about elective cessation: on the one hand, there is the hope that the disease and its arduous treatment will fade into the past; on the other is the fear of the child relapsing once he or she is no longer receiving chemotherapy. They question the wisdom of the child "not getting anything." While the child focuses more on the anticipated relief of being off treatment and not having to endure any more physical hardship, an element of ambivalence nonetheless lurks. Thus, the child and the parents must be reassured that elective cessation is both a crisis and a positive event and that fear and elation are its hallmarks.

RELAPSE

I am worried that something is going to happen to me again. I always
wish I had never had cancer in the first place. I *know* that I'm not going
to have cancer again. I *know* it.

A seven-year-old girl who was being investigated for the possibility of recurrence of her disease spoke these earnest words. Throughout the week of testing, she drew a series of vivid rainbows. Each
was placed centrally on the page, as a fulcrum between the sun on
one side and slashes of rain on the other (color plate XIII). The child
commented: "I don't know which side of the rainbow I'm on." Her
statement conveys the threat that relapse poses to the child and parents: a counterpoint to the hope for prolonged survival and cure.

Even a child too young to comprehend the precise implications
of the remission-relapse cycle is conscious of its existence. The child
who is undergoing, or has completed, active treatment, conceptual-
izes remission in such terms as "I have no more leukemia" or "the
disease has gone away." The fear of relapse is articulated as: "What if
I get sick again?" or "What if my disease comes back?" The child in-
tuitively understands that the disease could reassert itself, translating
the "possibility" of its presence into actuality.[21] While anxiety about
recurrence never entirely disappears, the intensity and pervasiveness
of the preoccupation do abate.

For a child in remission, triggers for anxiety about relapse include:
return visits to the clinic at regular intervals; physical symptoms, particularly those in any way associated with the diagnosis or treatment;
anniversary dates; and hearing of another patient's relapse or death.
The "follow-up" appointments in particular engender enormous
anxiety, especially if they include dreaded, painful procedures that
make explicit the ongoing vigilance for the recurrence of the disease.

The child's anxiety often starts to build days before the scheduled visit. It may manifest itself through direct statements ("What if they find the disease has come back?"), or indirectly through marked changes in behavior such as withdrawal, aggression, moodiness, or sleep disturbances. These effects reverse immediately once the child knows that everything is all right for another period of time.

What are the implications of relapse? In *most* instances, it indicates that treatment toward cure has failed and that the chances for the child's prolonged survival are diminished. While the caregivers experience a profound sense of sadness at this qualification of hope for the long-term future, they nonetheless harness their energy into planning the next treatment strategy. The parents must contend with a grief reaction reminiscent of the time of initial diagnosis, now complicated by the additional prognostic uncertainty that a relapse portends. Parents usually rally with an intensified determination to bring their child through this newest catastrophe. As one mother said: "When our child first got sick, we fought a battle to get him into remission. If he relapses now, after all this time, we'll fight a war." [22]

The emotional and lifestyle repercussions of relapse differ depending on when it occurs. A recurrence while still on the original treatment protocol usually represents the most serious blow to the child's chances for long-term survival. The parents' and caregivers' reactions reverberate intensely, whether or not the child clearly understands their meaning. On a day-to-day basis, however, the child may only experience the recurrence as the need for different medications or an alteration in schedule. Even if a hospitalization or more surgery is indicated, the child is still in the routine of the illness.

In contrast, the child who has been off treatment and "free" for a period of time, expresses outrage at the return of the illness. A sense of betrayal—by his or her body, by treatment, by the caregivers, even by the parents who once again have failed as protectors—is paramount. One question cuts straight through the anguish: "What will you do for me now?" The child recognizes the gravity of the situation and the need for action. The following interchange captures the immediacy:

Physician:　We've had a chance to look at your bone marrow and—
Jenny:　　　[interrupting] I'm not in remission anymore.
Physician:　Right. And you know that we want to discuss with you the possibility of doing a bone marrow transplant . . .
Jenny:　　　[immediately] I'll have it if that's my chance.

Terror at the prospect of returning to treatment, with a less salutary view of what the drugs can do, augments the child's sense of foreboding.

An eight-year-old boy, just prior to the confirmation of his relapse, reported a dream that ended: "He died inside." While he could not explain his dream further, the words bear ominous overtones of mortality.

In the weeks following an eleven-year-old girl's second relapse, she talked obsessively about all her pets who had died over the years. With the first recurrence of her disease, she had been matter-of-fact about going back on treatment. However, in the three-year interim, she had known several children who had relapsed and died. Thus, her current view incorporated an emotional and intellectual grasp of the seriousness of the implications.

The psychological tasks in adjusting to the relapse encompass both breadth and depth. At the most immediate level, the child may reexperience extreme difficulty in "getting used to" the physical hardship of the medical regimen. The rigors of treatment are much intensified by the fearful implications of the recurrence. Many children report a sense of battle fatigue, wherein their resilience in facing treatment has eroded and must be painstakingly reconstructed. The child must incorporate the clinic and hospital settings back into his or her life, while adjusting to the identity of being a patient once again. Challenges in facing the outer world, once thought to have been safely relegated to the past, must now be renegotiated. Most profound, the child must find renewed pathways toward hope for the future.

The physical and emotional terrors of the illness surge and recede over time. In a sea of uncertainty, the child's ongoing quest is to find a "safe place" within the storm. Initially, brief respite from aggressive treatment or hospitalization may suffice. Eventually, however, the child searches for the long-term safety of remission and, ultimately, of cure.

If kids are normal, not sick, they like to be treated special.
But if kids have a disease, they want to be treated normal.
(eleven-year-old girl)

"Longing for normalcy" is a refrain of many children after the diagnosis of a life-threatening illness. It is inextricably associated with time: the child refers to "normal" as how he or she was before the illness and hopes to be once again. However, life-threatening illness in a child is a profoundly *abnormal* phenomenon; its presence cannot be erased, nor its psychological effects reversed. "Normal" as a taken-for-granted presumption of daily life has been shattered by the diagnosis and its implications. Lenore Terr states: "Defenses go up very fast after trauma strikes. People do not wish to think of themselves as abnormal, hurt or changed.... It's not fair, they feel. And they are right—it's not fair.... But ... children's lives, 'normal' or 'abnormal,' may organize around a trauma."[1]

For the child, facets of "normal" include being regular (not special), ordinary (not exceptional), and fitting in (not being different). From looking to feeling to *being* normal, the concept has implications for the child's sense of competence and self-esteem.

The eleven-year-old girl quoted above continued: "Once you have a disease, people treat you as if you're not capable. Even though it's not true, it makes you feel really bad about yourself."

A seven-year-old girl intended to bake a birthday cake for her mother. However, when she came home from school, she found that her grandmother had already bought one. The girl was furious: "My grandmother said that she was just trying to help because she didn't think I'd be up to it. But I know when I'm too tired—this time I *was* up to it."

While secondary gains, such as gifts and attention, temporarily ease the child's duress, they cannot compensate for the pervasive hardship of the illness. Furthermore, the pleasure in these "extras" is mitigated by their attestation to the child's abnormal situation.

Karen wrote a story about having leukemia that included the following comment: "I have a friend who said she'd rather be sick and get presents than be well and healthy. But I'd give *anything* to be off treatment."

From the outset, learning to treat their child "as normally as possible" is a formidable task for parents, especially with regard to discipline. Yet, their ability to do so communicates a critical message to the child: while the *illness* is abnormal, he or she is still normal in their eyes. The parents' articulation of this belief (even when it is not always translated into action) provides the child with a foundation of confidence. As the child incorporates the routine of the illness and treatment into daily life, a new version of normalcy emerges. While not the same as "before the illness," the child nonetheless finds markers of stability within the altered reality. This is particularly true, of course, when treatment is successful.

The child who has been diagnosed at an early age, and treated over a long period of time, may know of no life other than illness. His or her own view of normalcy is shaped by this reality.

Jonathan: Did you have a lot of needles when you were six years old?
Therapist: No, I didn't.
Jonathan: Why not?

Therapist: Because I didn't have leukemia when I was six years old.
Jonathan: [matter-of-factly] Well, maybe you'll get it when you're grown up.[2]

Such a child certainly recognizes—and at times resents—being in a minority. However, the normalcy of the rest of the world is perceived to lie beyond his or her grasp.

A ten-year-old boy who had been treated almost continuously since the age of four sighed: "I just wish that I knew how it felt to be normal."

Whether the illness is a new or longstanding presence in the child's life, fearfulness is often a manifestation of its impact. The child who has navigated perilous waters in the medical environment is reluctant to approach anything in the outside world that is not obviously "safe." Terr refers to a "kind of panicky intensity that characterizes a traumatized child's fear of everyday things, of the 'mundane.'"[3]

Whereas fearfulness in a healthy child tends to be rooted in anxiety and is often transitory in nature, its origins for the ill child are in lived experience and can endure tenaciously. As if to counterbalance the terror, he or she retreats into extreme caution, taking neither initiatives nor chances. A pattern of avoidance and nonperformance develops within the confines of generalized constriction. Not surprisingly, the child's apprehensions in daily life often mask fears related to the illness. Following is an example of how a highly structured psychotherapeutic intervention can diminish this overlay, even when the core terror cannot be entirely assuaged.

An eleven-year-old girl was described by her parents as being extremely fearful. She had always tended to keep feelings to herself and rarely talked about her illness. Many years earlier, during long hospitalizations, the girl had ruminated about how children would get out of the hospital if there were a fire. Now she expressed concern about a fire breaking out at home. Her parents also noted that she was afraid to try anything new in her daily life and was even fearful of activities that she had once enjoyed. An example was her refusal to ride her bicycle. The girl acknowledged her fearfulness, admitting that its intensity puzzled her. Over four individual sessions, the therapist focused the discussion on her experiences with leukemia. At the beginning of each meeting, the girl drew a mandala to illustrate the following topics: "How it felt to have leukemia when I was much younger"; "How I feel now about having leukemia"; "How I felt when my friend died last year" (see color plate xxvi); and "How it felt last week to talk about my friend." What emerged through the process was her being "scared and worried" about another relapse. The girl requested a joint session with her parents, in which she explained her mandalas and disclosed her fears. In a follow-up meeting a month later, she reported that she was much less preoccupied with the leukemia and that she had not had the intrusive thoughts about fire. She had begun to ride her bicycle again.

Parents, in a parallel process to their child, also feel the effects of living with danger close at hand. Thus, an apprehensive child is often acting out the parents' anxieties as well as his or her own. While admonitions to "be careful" are usually necessary and reasonable, an intense overprotectiveness communicates fear. In response to the message always to stay within safe limits, the child draws demarcated lines, beyond which he or she will not venture.

When an eight-year-old girl was asked what changed after she got sick, her immediate response was: "I have to be more careful when I'm outdoors. My parents are always checking on me to make sure that I don't hurt myself."

While the fear originates in the child's experiences within the medical environment, its extent can vary widely. The further removed the dreaded situation is from the illness (in time and context), the more the trauma has overstepped its boundaries, intruding into the child's daily life.

Sometimes Poly Polar Bear gets scared at night and wakes me up. When he does that, I read him two stories and kiss him. (Ricky)

During the day, the child may "shadow" the parents constantly: a vigilance carried over from the hospital. Such fearfulness is acutely exacerbated in the dark of night, when all patients, regardless of age, report feeling the most alone. The child may sleep fitfully, with lights on and door open, and awaken frequently to come into the parents' room, eventually spending the entire night in their bed. Often parents are simply too exhausted to take the child back to his or her room. Furthermore, this arrangement may feel like a "solution" as much to the parents as to the child: togetherness counteracts the lurking fear of loss. For the child to sleep with the parents occasionally, especially during acute crises, is reasonable. Some dying children derive comfort from the constant presence of loved ones, through both their sleeping and waking hours. However, for the child who is *living* with the illness, the "occasional night" risks turning into a regular pattern. Over time, complications begin to emerge: the parents have no privacy or intimacy; the child's fearfulness has no chance to abate. Conflict develops.

Ricky absolutely refused to sleep in his own bed at home. To emphasize his stand even further, he began to refer to his bedroom as his "office," obviously the place one goes only in the daytime. During a hospitalization, he commented:

Ricky: Even though Daddy treats me a little bit bad, I still miss him.
Therapist: How does he treat you bad? What does he do?
Ricky: He doesn't let me sleep in his bed.

In a later hospitalization, he recounted a story in which "my bed busted."

Therapist:	Your bed busted! Have you been sleeping in your own bed at home?
Ricky:	No.
Therapist:	You've been sleeping with Mommy and Daddy?
Ricky:	[nodded matter-of-factly] So it doesn't matter if it busts.
Therapist:	Do you feel more comfortable sleeping with Mommy and Daddy?
Ricky:	[nodded]
Therapist:	What do you like better about sleeping with Mommy and Daddy than sleeping alone?
Ricky:	[stating the obvious] That I'm not alone!

A mother reported with exasperation and humor that she might as well throw out her birth control pills, since she and her husband never slept together any more without their four-year-old son between them. Ironically, the boy was an only child who was constantly asking his parents when they would have a baby. The mother finally used one issue to solve the other: she told the child that unless she and her husband could be together privately at night, there was not even a chance that he would have a younger brother or sister! Through discussion and negotiation, the boy eventually resumed sleeping in his own room.

The process of returning the child to his or her own bed can be frustrating and time-consuming. However, the child eventually gains an important sense of mastery in sleeping alone. Taking back control of the night is the child's victory.

FAMILY

I have a closer relationship with my family than most other kids because I've needed them more these last years.
(eleven-year-old boy)

My family and I have not been sleeping well lately.
(eight-year-old girl)

The child-in-the-family is a unit unto itself, with its own distinctive identity, strengths, and vulnerabilities. The child's ongoing struggle to withstand and integrate the trauma of life-threatening illness unfolds within this framework. His or her ability to cope is greatly influenced by the family—the individual and collective responses of its members. Under optimal circumstances, "the interior of the family assumes a central role in preserving the patient's psychological integrity."[4] The family affords a refuge in which the child can replenish psychic resources, shielded from the battering assault of the illness.

The myth that a child's life-threatening illness either unites or destroys a family reduces complexity to oversimplification. In fact, resilience or vulnerability to the stress of the illness depends upon a myriad of factors. A family's experience and means of coping with adversity in the past will, to some extent, predict its response in the present. Salient dimensions of family functioning, which must be viewed through a sociocultural as well as a psychological lens, include: open/closed style of communication (both informational and affective); close/distant emotional involvement; flexible/rigid roles; organized/chaotic overall structure. How power and control are defined and delegated within the family, as well as how children are viewed (in terms of their individualism and competence), must be understood. The availability of support from extended family, friends, and community is also an important consideration. Inextricably linked with all these variables are the nature and course of the disease itself. Certain factors severely compromise a family's capacity to adapt to the exigencies of a child's illness. For example, a history of psychiatric disturbance, marital conflict, addiction, abuse, and financial problems put a family at elevated risk.

Within a systems view, stress in one part of the family affects all the other members. Murray Bowen, a founder of family therapy, referred to the "emotional shock wave" phenomenon: "a network of underground 'aftershocks' of serious life events that can occur anywhere in the extended family system in the months or years following serious emotional events in a family. It occurs most often after the death or the *threatened death* [italics added] of a significant family member."[5] The child witnesses these reverberations and instinctively identifies his or her illness as the cause. Guilt is a common response, even in the rational light of knowing that he or she did not ask for the illness to happen.

An eleven-year-old girl reflected sadly: "My mother and father had a hard life. It's not that I think that it's my fault. There was nothing I could do about being sick. But it was like I was the last straw."

A four-year-old "only" child asked his parents: "Are you not having a new baby because you don't want another sick kid?"

A nine-year old boy had barely sat down before he began to speak: "I think that my illness causes problems for everybody. They all have to worry a lot. Last night when I'd already gone to bed, I heard my parents arguing about money. *They'd have enough money if I were dead.*" He burst into tears.

A ten-year-old girl listed each family member's reaction to her illness (excluding herself): "Mother—cried [sadness and anticipatory grief]; father—got thinner, but gained it back when I got better [psychosomatic expression]; brother—got uptight easily [chronic tension]; sister—got a boyfriend [peer support, or flight from pain in family]." The girl's cryptic descriptions portray the manifestations of stress in her family.

In many instances, the child denies that the illness has caused problems for the family. He or she may report positive changes, but is reluctant or unable to think of difficulties. It is as if the child cannot afford to acknowledge any stress because of the guilt associated with being its "cause."

In response to what had changed in her family, a twelve-year-old girl said: "To me, I couldn't see a change, although my family may have had to adjust themselves." She thus began with denial and then vaguely conceded that perhaps there was some impact.

From the outset, the child's definition of his or her "family" (both biological and psychological members), should be elicited. Without such information, the caregiver may make faulty assumptions of inclusion or exclusion and thus overlook valuable sources of support to the child. The nuclear family of child, siblings, and parents is at the core, surrounded by the extended family. In particular, grandparents frequently play a major role in the child's care. Close friends may be indistinguishable from "family," especially during crises. The child often names a pet as a family member—a relationship whose importance must not be underestimated. With the changing face of the structure of the family, latitude must be made for alternative and complicated arrangements. These include divorced and reconstituted (blended) families, with their inherent conflictual histories and new alliances; single-parent families; and children of gay parents. In families that have been ravaged by AIDS, the child may be orphaned while also living under the threat of his or her own death. Thus, in circumstances that range from the traditional to the extraordinary, the child's definition of "family" is a significant reality.

The presence of life-threatening illness, while linked most obviously to the ill child, creates changes in all the preexistent roles and relationships within the family. Most common is the intensification of the relationship between the child and the parents (especially the mother) and the exclusion of the healthy siblings. The centrality of attention accorded to the child is understandable, and even necessary, during critical periods. However, when this focus becomes the norm over time, a complicated tangle of dysfunction can result. The child wields too much power, the marital dyad is disrupted, and the siblings lose their visibility in the family. While the child often observes and worries about the imbalances incurred by the illness, his or her state of vulnerability and need overshadows these concerns. Furthermore, it is not the child's responsibility to redress the balance of the family constellation.

A six-year-old "only" child constantly tried to prevent his parents from going out on their own. He would predict terrible thunderstorms prior to their departure or have a temper tantrum when the babysitter arrived. When the therapist addressed the fact that parents need to spend time together, without kids, the boy responded: "See that window? I'm going to throw you out of it, and I'm going to handcuff my parents' hands together to a piece of furniture in here."

A nine-year-old girl explained: "I think that my brother and sister are really mad at me, because I get all the presents and a lot of attention. They think I'm spoiled. I'd be mad at me if I were them. But they don't have to go for treatments like I do."

If the child has functioned in some pivotal way in the family, his or her role may be dramatically affected by the onset of the illness.

A mother referred to her nine-year-old daughter as "our own family therapist." When the girl became sick, and thus unavailable for her usual role, her parents recognized how much they had relied on her to carry out their mandate.

The issue of "protection" within the family may emerge in various guises throughout the course of the illness. The child's anger that the parents were not able to keep him or her out of harm's way reflects a profoundly shaken sense of safety. Each time that the child encounters a new crisis or undergoes a painful procedure, the loss of protection is evoked anew. He or she learns early that parents are neither omnipotent nor invulnerable and that threatening forces operate even beyond their control. In witnessing the child's agony, the parents face their own helplessness.

In another facet of protection, the child tries to spare the parents the intensity of his or her fear and sadness. This stance is matched by the parents' attempts to shield the child from any further hardship, especially from witnessing *their* distress. Eventually a cycle is set in motion. This cycle isolates the child and parents from one another at exactly those times that mutual disclosure would create a comforting bridge.

Sibling relationships are a crucial axis in the family, a subsystem of their own.[6] Most children demonstrate an impressive capacity for concern about the siblings, although ambivalence intensifies under the stress of illness. Angry to be sick, the child resents the brothers and sisters for their health. Protests of injustice ("it's not fair that I got sick and he didn't") bring only short-lived relief, followed by remorse. Inextricable with this anger is the child's guilt at his or her "monopoly" on the parents' time and energy. It is not unusual for a child to declare that a brother or sister has been a "best friend" through the hardship. He or she discovers a new appreciation for the siblings' abiding presence and companionship. To ignore the potential richness of this relationship is to neglect an invaluable resource for the child.

The family holds the child tight within its arms, braced against the threat of the illness. It is from this base that he or she ventures into the world of school and peers.

SCHOOL

School is the defining structure of every child's day-to-day life. More than any other activity, it represents constancy, a routine with a stable set of rules and expectations. Erik Erikson referred to the developmental task of the school-aged child as "industry versus inferiority," the striving for competence and self-worth garnered from achievements and investments in the world of school and peers.[7] If the child's functioning is compromised, particularly over an extended period of time, he or she may be vulnerable to a diminished sense of self-esteem.

In the past, the child with a life-threatening illness was simply tutored in the hospital setting or at home. Now that children live longer, or are eventually cured, prompt reintegration into the classroom after the initiation of treatment is pivotal. For the child whose routine has been wrested away by the intrusion of the illness, school becomes the normalizing axis of daily life. Far from the harrowing world of the medical center and the intensity of the family, it provides a safe environment for learning and mastery.

Karen emphasized the importance of academic accomplishment in her family drawing. She portrayed herself exuberantly as "Karen the Great," wearing a kerchief on her head, grinning broadly, and brandishing an A+ report card (figure 24). Furthermore, of all the outfits in Snoopy's wardrobe that she had just begun to collect, it was his cap and gown for graduation that she wanted most urgently.

The return to school is a milestone for both child and parents, especially as it follows the emotional fusion of the diagnostic period. As with any new threshold, there is ambivalence: the eagerness to

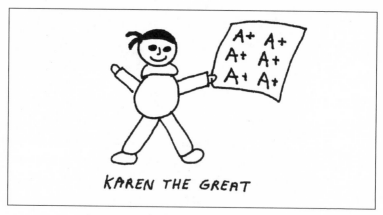

FIGURE 24. *A+ report card*

venture out is counterbalanced by the fear of separation. The child must reenter the world on his or her own; the parents must relinquish their proximity and vigilance. Understandably, the parents' support to the child is often given *despite* their own anxiety. Yet, it is their readiness that enables the child's successful return.

As in many aspects of the illness experience, it is important that the child exert a measure of control in the preparation for reentry. Thus, the child may have specifications about what the school personnel should, or should not, know about his or her condition. When parents and caregivers provide information, it relieves the child of the burden of explanation, to whatever extent he or she chooses.

A twelve-year-old boy wrote the following message prior to the medical team's visit to his school: "Please stress the fact that I am no longer sick, but in remission and receiving treatment. Thanks." In the margin, he had sketched part of a tree trunk, with an offshoot of new leaves unfolding. This depiction of life emphasized the boy's request to focus on his return to health, rather than on the illness alone (figure 25).

The child benefits from rehearsal on how to answer questions, dispel rumors, and deal with difficult interpersonal situations that may arise. Fearful that social ostracism may be compounded by lags in academic performance, he or she often requests remedial help prior to the return to school, if not on an ongoing basis.

Preparation of the professionals in the school to reintegrate the child is the essential counterpoint of the process. Educating the school nurse is necessary, but not sufficient. It is the teacher who becomes the child's caregiver for the better part of each day and who may initially be quite frightened by that responsibility. Thus, he or she must have access to information concerning the child's illness and an opportunity to voice questions, concerns, and apprehensions. The counselors and administrators, who provide a support network for both the child and teacher, must also be well informed.

Many medical centers now offer education and consultation to

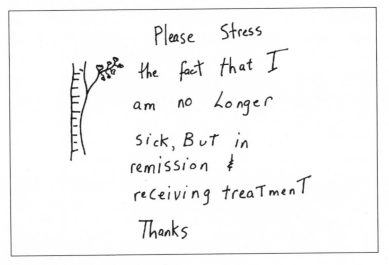

FIGURE 25. *I am no longer sick*

school personnel, either on a programmatic or an individual basis. Workshops afford a valuable forum for introducing these professionals to medical and psychological aspects of the illness. Topics to highlight include: a basic understanding of the disease and modalities of treatment, physical side effects, behavioral or mood changes, impact on attention and learning, and the emotional reverberations of the illness on the child and family. Myths about the contagion of disease must be dispelled; in reality, it is the *patient* who may have to be protected from many of the common infectious illnesses of childhood. Interwoven with these topics is guidance on how best to be sensitive to the ill child, what to anticipate from the other students, and how to handle their reactions. An organized tour of the medical center instills invaluable empathy for the child's experience in his or her "other world." Printed resource material consolidates the learning and can be distributed to those staff members not present at the workshop. The contact between the treatment team and the school personnel at these meetings establishes a liaison that endures throughout the child's illness.

A conference with school personnel to focus on an individual child is important, whether or not a workshop program is in place. Many parents feel comfortable in setting up such a meeting on their own, with the treatment team as backup. For others, who may be distant or even alienated from the school system, the medical center team must take the initiative. Factors such as geographical distance, or the school's past experience with an ill child, also influence the extent of the team's direct involvement.

The opportunity for classmates to learn about the illness and express their concerns before the ill child's return to school is crucial. If their anxiety is assuaged, hurtful confrontations can be minimized. The fact that classmates' occasional cruelty arises out of a sense of threat is small comfort to the child who suffers under wounding comments or stares.

An eight-year old girl had gone to Disneyworld, sponsored by a foundation that grants wishes to seriously and terminally ill children. On her return, she was furious to see an article about her trip in the town newspaper. Both her leukemia and the foundation were mentioned in some detail. In a letter berating the journalist, the girl dictated: "I didn't like you putting my personal business in the paper. You wrote that I have leukemia. Everyone thinks you're going to die when they read that, because years ago they didn't have medicines. Now they'll probably think I'm going to die." The girl's apprehensions were realized. In her first week back at school, a boy approached her to say that he had heard that she was going to die. She then had a series of recurrent nightmares of children forming a circle around her chanting: "You're going to die."

The child who has made a good adjustment back to school resents missing any more time. However, absences are an intrinsic part of ongoing medical treatment. Between school and the medical center, the child is actually running on two full-time schedules, each with its own set of demands. Thus, he or she always feels the need to "catch up" with something happening at school. Compounding the absences is fatigue, a factor that pervades the child's day-to-day functioning while still on treatment.

A seven-year-old girl was being investigated for the possibility of a recurrence. The focus of her anxiety was missing school: "Will the teacher count the days I'm absent if I have a relapse?"

Karen reported on Poly Polar Bear, following her own return to school: "He liked being back, but he's exhausted by all the work."

The establishment of reasonable criteria for performance is a challenge for both child and teacher. On the one hand, clear expectations are necessary for the child to feel involved in the learning process and to be part of the class. On the other hand, the rigors of the illness and treatment regimen, ongoing absences, fatigue, and emotional stress must all be taken into account. The onus is on the teacher to recognize these factors, to be patient, and to respect the child's competence and dignity in the process. Even with the best of intentions, striking a balance between rigidity and flexibility is not easy. Errors in judgment can result in the child feeling discouraged and inadequate at a time when he or she can least afford these reactions.

A nine-year-old boy had received only sporadic tutoring during a long absence. In his first week back at school, tests were scheduled in several subjects. Despite the child's protests, the teacher insisted that he write them with the class. While she intended to use his results simply as a guide for remediation, the boy was devastated by his poor performance. "She should have just talked to me about what I had missed," he explained. "That way, I wouldn't have felt so bad about not knowing anything."

Karen, always a high achiever, reported a shift in her parents' expectations of her academic performance: "They always told me to do my best. Now they're saying it's okay not to get A's, but I don't believe them." When Karen entered fifth grade, the school placed her in the regular stream, instead of honors, hoping to reduce any extra pressure. However, Karen responded with bitterness: "I feel deprived—punished by my illness—to be taken out of honors." After consultation with her parents, Karen was returned to the more demanding program.

A seven-year-old boy who had been out of school for most of first grade was promoted at the end of the year. He was outraged: "That stupid principal! Why did he pass me? I don't even know how to read yet. They just did it because they feel sorry for me."

When a child's treatment goes well, the initial diagnostic period may be his or her only prolonged absence from school. However, for many children, reentry is not a singular event. While the first return is often the hardest, since there has been no precedent, subsequent returns must be planned with the same care if they are to be successful. In certain circumstances, later reentries may prove even more difficult. For example, a child whose disease recurs off treatment, after a period of looking and feeling normal, may find the return to school after the reinitiation of therapy an exceedingly vulnerable undertaking.

Another example of this problem arises when a child changes schools, after having accomplished the initial return in a familiar setting. He or she enters not only as "the new kid" but as "the new kid who is sick." Many children who have completed treatment choose not to talk about their past medical history with classmates, even when it is recent. In some ways, the child uses the change of schools to mark a new chapter, free from the illness. Any disclosure must be left to his or her discretion.

An eight-year-old boy did not divulge anything of his past illness until the school mounted a fund-raising drive for "his" medical center. At that point, he decided to speak up in order to make the campaign more meaningful for the other students. He described all the things that are done to help sick children become well again, and concluded: "I'm the proof!"

Entering school for the first time—either nursery or kindergarten—is always a challenging threshold to cross. For the child who has lived traumatic separation experiences in the context of illness, the prospect can be even more daunting.

A three-year-old boy had had long hospitalizations during his eighteen-month illness. Nonetheless, he went fairly willingly to his first day of nursery school. At the end of the day, the teacher reported to his mother: "He only wanted to take one shoe off for rest-time today, but that was fine. Perhaps next time he'll be ready to take off both shoes. We thought it was great that he would trust us halfway!" The teacher's sensitivity to the boy's extraordinary past experience allowed him a gradual adjustment to the routine, without forcing him to drop his guard too quickly.

There are always individual, idiosyncratic problems that cannot be foreseen. It is for exactly this reason that ongoing communication among the school personnel, parents, and caregivers is so important.

The three-year-old boy did well in group activities at nursery school. However, when taken aside individually for speech therapy, he became upset, agitated, and inattentive. In discussion with the psychologist, his mother realized that the boy's only past experience of intensive "one-on-one" had been the physician examining him. Once this fearful parallel was recognized, the speech therapist was able to engage him gradually through play.

An eight-year-old boy came home in a panic: "We're going to have *tests* in school tomorrow." His understanding of "tests" was of painful, medical procedures; he had had no other experience of the word. During the same year, the boy's teacher noted that he was too voluble in class discussions. His mother explained that for five years, his "talking doctor" had encouraged him to express his feelings and that it would be hard for him to change his habits now!

The disease itself or a treatment modality (e.g., central nervous system radiation) may permanently affect a child's cognitive functioning. The effects may be immediate or delayed in specific areas of learning, or in behavior. Common behavioral disorders include deficits in attention or impulse control. Whatever the nature of the impairment, precise neuropsychological assessment and ongoing remediation are crucial.

School avoidance is a disabling psychological reaction that represents *extreme* separation difficulties shared by parent and child, although its manifestation is in the child's behavior. In the absence of any medical prohibition, he or she refuses to attend school. The reality-based fears of separation, intrinsic to life-threatening circumstances, are elaborated into an immobilizing overlay of anxiety. School avoidance thus emerges as a symptom in and of itself. It may present explicitly, in verbal protests and tantrums, or indirectly, through somatic complaints. Parents have a difficult time ignoring or overruling physical symptoms, especially those in any way associated with the illness. Unfortunately, school avoidance is often minimized—or not reported at all—until it has escalated to crisis proportions. In such instances, intensive psychotherapy may be necessary to enable the child's return. Caregivers' awareness of the risk for school avoidance in seriously ill children fosters an atmosphere of prevention, whereby ongoing monitoring of attendance is built into the overall treatment plan.

Early in the illness, the home and hospital are the child's major points of reference, with school in the background. Over time, the medical center's omnipresence recedes, and school reemerges as the familiar context for the developmental tasks of childhood.

PEERS

Peer relationships are a source of validation for all children. Within the context of a life-threatening illness, friendships provide crucial support and enhancement of a child's sense of self-worth. It is not uncommon for the child to develop two categories of friends: those from the "healthy" world of school and neighborhood, and those from the hospital, clinic, and specialized camps for children with similar illnesses.

The child often expresses apprehension about the anticipated re-action of his or her peers: how will they tolerate "differentness"? Will the child be accepted, or will he or she be teased, stigmatized, reject-ed? Who will remain steadfast through difficult times ahead? The child fears that "friends from before" (an expression frequently used) will withdraw out of fear, impatience, or simply not knowing how to approach.

A nine-year-old boy reflected: "At first my friends seemed afraid of me. They were trying to act as if nothing was different, but I could tell that they didn't know what to say. I didn't know what to say either. Except I wanted to remind them that I was still the same kid as before, even if I looked different."

True friends are clearly distinguished from those whose loyalties waver or evaporate once the illness has struck. Most children report that some friends have stood by them, albeit often with hurt and misunderstandings along the way. The difficulties usually revolve around feeling left out of the network of activities or shared confi-dences.

An eight-year-old girl was hurt that she had not been invited to a class-mate's birthday party. She decided to confront her friend about the ex-clusion. "My friend just said: 'You're always sick. I just didn't think you'd be able to come.' I told her that I would have felt better if she had at least asked me."

Peers who make overtures for the first time in the period after the diagnosis are often met with wariness: the child suspects that pity or curiosity has fueled their interest. Over time, the child gradually de-velops a highly attuned sense of the motivation of others in initiat-ing friendship.

Some children, in an almost counterphobic way, convert what could be the stigma of the illness into a badge of courage and fascination. In effect, they reframe their differentness from that of victim into that of hero. Many choose to do a school project or presentation on their illness and treatment. By explaining the experience, the child extends a bridge of candor toward his or her peers.

A ten-year-old girl reported: "My friends were great! They sent me lots of cards when I was in the hospital and phoned me when I got home. When I came back to school, I asked them to help me with the work I had missed. I explained my treatments to them—they couldn't believe what I have to go through. . . . My best friend wanted to see my bald head. She even thought it looked kind of cool!"

Parents can play a pivotal role in facilitating the development or resumption of their child's peer relationships. They may collaborate actively with the child or advocate "behind-the-scenes" with other parents, teachers, and recreational leaders in the community. Such support is particularly important for the child who is reluctant to take the risk of initiating social contact after the diagnosis. When difficult or hurtful peer interactions occur, parents must be prepared to see the child through to a resolution, despite the intensity of their own fiercely protective or angry reactions.

The relationships that develop through the hospital and clinic are of a different nature. United as "comrades" by the illness experience, staunch friendships arise in the absence of other commonalities and despite differences that would have ordinarily separated the children. The child often comments that other patients are the only ones who truly understand what he or she has endured.

A seven-year-old boy reported feeling "kind of good" when he heard that there were other children in his community with cancer. "I didn't feel good because they had cancer. I just felt good because I didn't feel so alone anymore."

There has been, and in some medical centers continues to be, controversy about whether children with life-threatening illnesses should all be hospitalized on one unit or distributed throughout the general pediatric population. Increasingly, they are grouped together, both to facilitate the medical treatment and in recognition of the unique support network that develops among the children and parents. Natalie Kusz remembers her own experience:

We found it both interesting and difficult enough to keep current daily record of who had been examined, tested, or operated upon, and whether it had hurt, and if so, whether they had cried. This last question was always of interest, and tears we looked on as marks, not of cowards, but of heroes, playmates who had endured torture and lived to testify.... Those of us who did choose to abide vigorously in each instant were able to offer ourselves, during the day, to one another, to uphold that child or parent who began to weaken. If her need was to laugh, we laughed together; if to talk, we listened; and once, I remember, I stood a whole morning by the chair of a fifteen-year-old friend, combing her hair with my fingers, handing her Kleenex and lemon drops, saying nothing.[8]

Structured self-help groups can provide a forum for children to share experiences in living with serious illness. However, the threat and impact of loss are amplified once a cohesive group forms. Thus, facilitators must be trained to respond to such eventualities.

Over the last decade, summer camps have been established specifically for children with life-threatening illnesses. These programs afford the child a sense of belonging, the comfort of being in the majority, instead of in a tiny minority of the wider world. Self-consciousness about any limitation or handicap is erased in the recognition that all the children have been through similar trials.

An eleven-year-old girl thought it might be "weird" to attend a camp for children with cancer. However, she returned home enthusiastic: "It was still like a regular camp, with activities and bunks and counselors. But nobody there felt different. Nobody had to wear a kerchief or hat if they didn't feel like it. We were all going through the same things with treatment and everything. I just hope that all the friends I met will be okay when I go back next summer."

Wherever these friendships among patients develop—medical center, support group, or camp—the threat of loss lurks at the periphery. In this shadow, a spectrum of styles of attachment is evident. At one end are children who shy away from closeness to others in precarious circumstances; at the other are those who form intense and vigilant relationships with other patients.

Soon after her own diagnosis, Karen had had a terminally ill roommate in the hospital. She thus learned early and shockingly of the course the illness could take. From that time on, Karen seldom asked about other patients, and kept her distance from them while in the clinic or hospital. Even in the playroom, she tended to immerse herself in individual projects. In fact, Poly Polar Bear functioned as her closest "peer" in the medical setting.

Jenny kept in close touch with several other patients. At one point she informed the therapist about a little boy she had seen that morning in the clinic: "He's not doing well. That's about it—but that's a lot." Once in remission, and only coming to the clinic at much longer intervals, Jenny would phrase her questions about acquaintances as: "Is ———— still alive?"

The child's proclivity for relationships with other patients must be respected, although extremes can be troubling. A child's reluctance to make any contact may signal difficulty in assimilating the illness into his or her identity. (This reaction is, however, quite normal in a child who is newly diagnosed and has not yet absorbed all that has happened.) On the other hand, a child whose emotional energy is overwhelmingly invested in other sick children begins to live in a universe constricted by illness and loss. Most children eventually achieve a balance between their involvement and concern toward other patients and their maintenance of a foothold in the world of the healthy, to which they aspire to return.

The impact of the illness on the child's daily life—family, school, and peers—is pervasive. Within these intertwined spheres, the child pursues the pathways of "ordinary" existence—a version of normalcy revised by extraordinary circumstance.

✄ Facets of Awareness

A five-year-old child explained the Medic Alert bracelet that he wore (indicating that he was on chemotherapy): "It's for in case I sink. It can help people get me out of the water—like a lifesaver."

My mother's friend has cancer. She's getting experimental chemo, like me. You know—no guarantees. *(Jenny)*

The child's awareness of the life-threatening implications of the illness can be conceptualized along a continuum.[1] At one end, the child acknowledges being "very sick" or having a "bad disease"; however, there is no prognostic statement referring to life or death. In the middle, the child expresses some awareness that his or her life might be in jeopardy—uncertainty about *living*—but without a focus on death. At the other end of the continuum, the child is explicitly conscious that he or she could die of the illness. Awareness is gleaned from many sources. Primary is the "wisdom of the body": the child's irrefutable recognition of how sick he or she is. Other cues include the child's knowledge of the illness, the urgency and intensity of treatment, the emotions of family and caregivers, and encounters with other patients. Awareness is a fluid, not a static state. Thus, dependent on current medical status, or related to a significant life event, the child's comments and play will incorporate different elements at different times. The therapist must be highly attuned to the child's level of consciousness; otherwise he or she will negate or cut off the communication.

Karen overheard her mother talking to another parent about bone marrow transplantation being a "risky procedure." Karen broke in and asked: "You mean kids can still die from leukemia?" Later that week, she confided to the therapist that she was worried about the child who was undergoing the transplantation and scared for herself. When the therapist asked her if she was ever frightened about dying, she retorted loudly: "I'M NOT WORRIED ABOUT THAT."

The following drawings attest to the child's awareness of vulnerability, with and without verbal disclosure.

An eleven-year-old girl reported having seen a television interview of a teenager who had had her leg amputated. "She said that she would have died without the amputation. I guess my medicines are like her amputation." The child then showed the therapist a drawing that she had done secretly in school that day: a cobblestone walk leads up to a tombstone on which the words "Here Lies Nobody" are inscribed (figure 26). She giggled anxiously in handing over the picture and could not

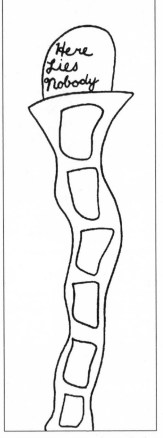

FIGURE 26. *Here lies nobody*

explain it except to say that it was "a joke." However, in light of her comment about her medicines, its significance could not be underestimated.

A seven-year-old girl reported: "Even my cats are worried about me. They sleep on my bed. And my dog—he doesn't sleep on my bed, but he stays in my room." She then drew a picture of her house which elaborated her sense of foreboding and vulnerability (color plate xiv). It is black, with a dark brown roof and tiny windows. The outside staircase is an unstable zigzag that is not anchored to the ground. A driveway stops short of the house. All the apples on the tree are in the process of falling or have already fallen into the grass.

Jenny drew a walnut for Nutty the Squirrel: a pronounced crack, like a fault line in the earth, bisects it (color plate xv). Another nine-year-old girl, for whom trees had been her "lifeline," began to draw them with gaping black holes in the trunks. The holes are so large that, in fact, they sever the trees. A small bird sits precariously high in the foliage (color plate xvi). In both drawings, a symbolic "flaw" figures prominently.

The child's awareness is expressed in both cognitive and emotional terms. Comments may be phrased quite matter-of-factly or cloaked in allusion. Whatever their form, they indicate the thought that the child has given to his or her life status. Questions or statements of medical fact do not belie the enormous emotion that pervades the topic; however, intellectualization can be a crucial defense and means of coping for the child.

The young child, in a way that is developmentally appropriate, is curious about the distinction between being alive and being dead. There may not be any form of self-reference explicitly expressed in this interest. However, at a fundamental level, consciously or not, the child is grappling with the concepts that have become salient with the onslaught of the illness. The theme of "alive-dead" may recur in an almost ritualized form as the child attempts to work through his or her comprehension.

Jonathan picked up a bottle containing many tiny shells that the therapist kept on her desk. In great excitement he exclaimed: "I think they're alive! I saw one move! They store their own food and water. Maybe they even have a sink in there!" After his session, he told the child life specialist about the shells and asked her opinion as to whether or not they were alive.

Ricky was desperately trying to understand how Johnny, a three-year-old child on the ward, had died. The therapist recognized that Ricky might better understand "dead" if he could conceptualize "alive." Thus, she asked: "Do you know what it means to be alive? What are some of the things that we can do because we are alive?" Together, Ricky and the therapist listed and played out different actions; for example, walk, talk, look, sing, jump on the bed. The activities were done with great enjoyment and elaboration. At the end, the therapist concluded: "These are all things that we can do when we are alive. When we are dead, we can't do them anymore." In the next session, Ricky talked about shooting the monsters in his dreams. The therapist asked: "You kill the monsters so that they're dead?" Ricky responded: "What is dead? Can they walk and run?" The therapist then proceeded to play the alive-dead distinction game with him again. A week later, Ricky reported that "Poly Polar Bear doesn't understand the point of it." When the therapist asked Ricky what he meant, he answered: "The point of it—like dead—what is dead?" This was his invitation to play the game. At the end of three weeks, Ricky had consolidated the concepts:

Therapist: When we're alive, what kind of things can we do?
Ricky: Move, hit, punch, see, walk.
Therapist: You can do lots of things when you're alive, right?
Ricky: Uh-huh.
Therapist: And what happens when you die? What does it mean?
Ricky: You don't do any of those things. Your heart stops beating.

Whether or not the child has talked about his or her own situation directly, a heightened sensitivity to issues of life and death is often evident. This form of awareness may express itself in an outburst, which, under ordinary circumstances, might be judged as an overreaction. However, it is often these very episodes, unpredictable in their occurrence, that demonstrate the child's vulnerability.

A three-year-old boy overheard his mother talking about a neighborhood child who had been hurt in an accident. He began chanting: "I no die. You no die. Daddy no die. Brothers and sisters no die. Brownie [family dog who had been given away] die."

A seven-year-old boy accidentally knocked a friend off his bicycle. The friend teasingly "played dead" for a few seconds and then stood up. The panicked boy ran into the house, crying to his mother: "How could he do that to me if he's my best friend?"

Some children develop a theory of their illness that protects them against the full awareness of its life-threatening nature. Such explanations may involve careful reasoning, "logical" rationalization, or even outright denial. Whatever their form—often a combination of all the elements—these carefully constructed defenses must be respected.

A four-year-old boy insisted on watching a leukemia telethon in its entirety "because it's about 'kemia.'" Soon thereafter, he expressed his belief that "*only* kids [he was an only child] don't die because then their parents wouldn't have any kids. . . . Kids only die if they have brothers and sisters." Two months later the boy stated: "I don't have 'kemia.' Everyone says I do, but I just fell down the stairs. Because you die if you have 'kemia.'" In fact, pain and weakness in his legs had been his presenting symptoms, and he had fallen down the stairs.

Ricky spontaneously offered his theory of what is necessary for life. His confidence that he himself could fulfill that definition increased as the dialogue progressed. His initial doubt about food reflected the fact that he was not eating very much at the time.

Ricky: We can only live with meat, which is food and ... toys and love.

Therapist: Food, toys, and love are what we need. Do you think that you've got all those things? Do you have food?

Ricky: Yah [somewhat dubiously].

Therapist: Enough? Do you think you have enough food?

Ricky: Yah!

Therapist: Toys?

Ricky: Uh-huh. Look! [He pointed to all his stuffed animals.]

Therapist: How about love? Who loves you?

Ricky: Mommy, Daddy, all the nurses and my doctor. Do you love me?

Therapist: I do love you.

Ricky: So everyone here loves me. ...

Therapist: You've got lots of love.

Ricky's definition was a profound truth for him. Almost three months later, with no mention of it in the interim, he repeated his belief verbatim. Even the doubtful quality of enough food remained in his reference to "running out of it."

Therapist: Do you remember the three things you said you need to live?

Ricky: Food, toys, and love.

Therapist: Do you have any more to add now?

Ricky: Uh-huh. Meat. Juice. Breakfast.

Therapist: Do you think you have enough food these days?

Ricky: When they run out of it, they can just go out and buy more.

Therapist: How about toys?

Ricky: Everyone just goes out and buys me some.

Therapist: How about love? Who loves you?

Ricky: Everyone. And I know you do.

A child may state quite matter-of-factly that he or she has been near death. Such frank acknowledgment often emerges once the child is better and knows that he or she is out of danger. The conscious awareness that death could have actually occurred may be based upon a single episode or upon the broader implications of the diagnosis. This type of reflection is distinct from that of the *dying* child, who is living the reality of imminent death. In the following series of vignettes, the spectrum ranges from responses in the immediate aftermath of a crisis, to a more pensive, retrospective view of having outlived death. The children's candor and accuracy are stunning.

During the previous night, Ricky's temperature and blood pressure had dropped precipitously. Although he was revived quickly, he had been blue, hard to rouse, and very cold. He looked gray and peaked the next day, when the following conversation took place.

Therapist: What do the nurses do for you in the isolation room?
Ricky: Take my temperature, listen to my heart … and … my blood pressure.
Therapist: They check your blood pressure. Has it been okay lately?
Ricky: Yah. … It wasn't too good last night.
Therapist: It wasn't? What happened last night?
Ricky: Well, I almost died.
Therapist: You almost died? What happened, Ricky?
Ricky: Well, my temperature was down … my blood pressure was down … my heart was down. …
Therapist: Really! Were you scared?
Ricky: Yah—but I'm still alive!

At the end of the session, Ricky asked to listen to the tape. When he heard himself say: "But I'm still alive!" he exclaimed: "Thank God!" Later in the session, Ricky had reported that: "Poly Polar Bear is very sad now because he didn't swim. The water was ice." Through this image of Poly and the ice water, Ricky reiterated his own traumatic experience of being "cold."

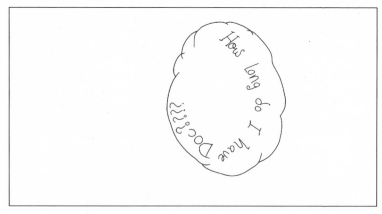

FIGURE 27. *How long do I have, Doc?*

During a particularly difficult hospitalization, Karen stated: "Last night, I felt as if I wouldn't make it through the night."

An eleven-year-old girl reported: "Many times in the bone marrow transplant room I came close to dying, but I didn't know it then."

A seven-year-old boy recounted: "My grandpa had cancer. He died last year. I could have died from my cancer, but I was lucky."

Drawings also attest to the child's explicit awareness of the threat of death. The following pictures all reflect a "scariest" image.

A twelve-year-old girl recounted: "When I first heard my diagnosis, one question kept going around and around in my head: 'How long do I have?' But I was too afraid to ask" (figure 27). In the next drawing (figure 28), a ten-year-old boy depicted a skull and crossbones leering above a bone marrow aspiration needle. In figure 29, an eleven-year-old boy portrayed himself lying in a hospital bed, the finality of death symbolized in his thoughts of a tombstone.

Other facets of the child's awareness are revealed in his or her perceptions of time, remembered dreams, and spiritual views.

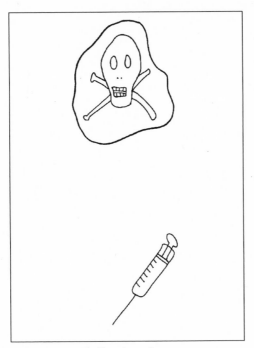

FIGURE 28. *Skull and crossbones*

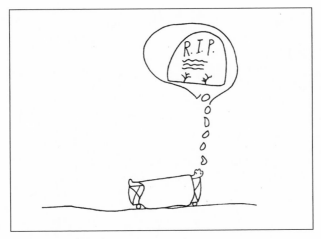

FIGURE 29. *Tombstone*

TIME

It takes a lot of days to be grown up, doesn't it? (Jonathan)[2]

The experience of life-threatening illness acutely heightens the child's awareness of time. The diagnosis ruptures the continuity between past and present, as if a bold line has severed the flow. In living "through" the present, the child's quest is for a seamless transition into the future. Yet the journey is fraught with uncertainty, wherein time holds no guarantees. This inability to take time for granted during childhood represents a crucial loss of innocence.

The child's temporal allusions may be direct, indirect, or metaphorical; matter-of-fact or tinged with sadness and anxiety. Whatever their form, time has emerged as a highly salient dimension in the child's life.

Of the thirty-five outfits shown in an illustrated catalogue of Snoopy's wardrobe, Karen had annotated the thirty-one that she did not yet have. Two of the outfits were marked "at the gift shop," a reference to the cancer center which was so much a part of her life. *All* of the other annotations referred to time! Her notes about when to buy each outfit (written above each picture) were as follows: "anytime" (six outfits); for a particular season (twelve); "year round" (four); "for graduation—right away when first see it!" (one); "for special occasions" (three); "if he's going to Japan, China, Hong Kong or France—anytime if not" (two). The last outfit in the catalogue ended on a poignant note: "hopefully soon."

A four-year-old boy coveted the child life specialist's Mickey Mouse watch. He tried it on, inspected it from every angle on his wrist, and said: "I like time. I wish I could wear a whole armful of watches." Later that day, in describing the watch to the therapist, he sighed: "I just wish that I had armfuls of time."

Even before the child has developed a precise cognitive sense of time, a global awareness of the tenses—past, present, and future—

exists. Although the tenses always overlap to some extent, it is possible to examine the child's references to time in each category.

Of the Past

While childhood should be lived in the present and the future, reflecting on the past is an important part of integrating experience. Once a child has been diagnosed with a life-threatening illness, the past takes on a power—and a vulnerability—all its own.

A focus on the past often represents a longing for the time before the illness, when life was still "normal." Not infrequently, a child may show the caregivers a photograph taken before the diagnosis, as if to say: "This is how I *really* look." Or, a child may describe past accomplishments, which, at least temporarily, seem out of reach. While the past certainly evokes sadness, it also serves positively as an impetus for "return." When a child resumes former activities, or removes a hat to show off newly growing hair, the past has triumphed in its reemergence in the present.

Quite often, the diagnosis of a life-threatening illness thrusts even the recent past into remoteness. Anything preceding the state of being ill recedes in the intensity of the present.

A six-year-old boy who had been diagnosed only a few months earlier, stated: "I don't know how I got sick. It was a very long time ago." In a similar testimony, an eight-year-old girl, whose father had died a year before her diagnosis, reported: "I don't remember when my father died. I was only a kid when he died."

Even more striking in some children is how the past vanishes into oblivion after the diagnosis. It is as if the child's entire memory has been conquered and inhabited by the illness, blocking access to the past. A child's claim to have forgotten everything attests to the overwhelming trauma engendered by the diagnosis. In part, this "forgetting" may be a defense against the pain of remembering a happier time. Eventually, as life redresses its balance, some of these children will reclaim earlier memories.

A ten-year-old girl stated: "I don't remember anything from before I got sick. I was so sick during the transplant that it just wiped everything else out."

A nine-year-old boy recounted that his one memory from before the diagnosis (at age six) was of being drowsy in the family's orchard. While in the hospital, he could calm his anxiety only by rocking slowly in a rocking chair. Through the soothing motion, he seemed able to return to that remembered drowsiness, when he had been healthy.

Perspectives on the past differ, depending upon the individual child, the age at diagnosis, and the trajectory of the illness. A gradual reconstruction of the past is crucial in the child's finding his or her place in time.

In the Present

In the same way that the future seemed, because it might never arrive, generally less important than the present, so, too, with the past. Although each of us children could have recited his own case history by heart, it was rare that any of us required more than a faint sketch of another child's past.[3]

The present tense is a hallmark of the child's experience in the medical world. Treatments are begun *now* on a strict schedule. The child picks up a sense of the immediacy, if not the urgency, of time in this environment. An unusually dramatic instance of this collapsing of time into the present is evident in the following vignette:

Jenny knew that she would be entering the bone marrow transplant room "soon." One morning, her physician informed her: "We have to move faster on the transplant than we had thought." Visibly shaken, Jenny asked: "You mean like in two days or a week?" The physician replied: "No, like *tonight* you move into the room." In the next few minutes, Jenny had to assimilate her projection of future time into the immediate present.

For the seriously ill child, it is only the present that can offer reassurance, a reliability that the future may not hold. Without actually knowing such credos as "one day at a time," or "make today count," many children instinctively focus on the present in their adaptation to uncertainty.

An eight-year-old boy reported: "The doctors think my bone marrow is fine for now—and *for now* is *for now*."[4]

An eleven-year-old girl drew an animated family picture, portraying herself as a skating instructor for younger children. When asked what changed in the family after she got sick, she wrote: "The whole family changed, and we don't plan ahead like we used to. We live each day as it comes" (figure 30).

The child's functioning in-the-moment pervades daily life beyond the medical setting. Parents convey the sense of a child who packs everything in, leaving nothing for later. The "now" becomes paramount. The mother of an eight-year-old child commented: "My son is not casual about life." She explained that everything seemed to have a clarity of purpose for him, so unlike the meanderings that ordinarily typify childhood.

Impatience is often observed and reported. For a healthy child, the feeling of being unable to wait expresses pleasurable anticipation. In illness, waiting is more often fraught with anxiety. Lurking at some level is the fear that something bad will happen to prevent the child from reaching the goal.

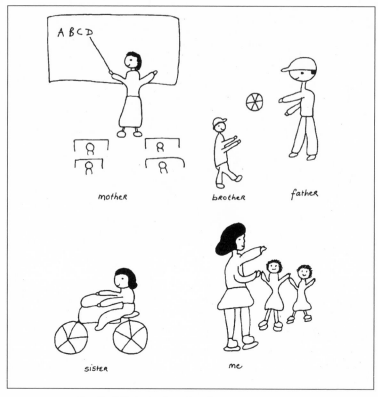

FIGURE 30. *Family: We don't plan ahead*

Karen commented playfully: "Poly Polar Bear is very impatient. He's the imp and I'm the patient!" It is as if impatience defines the very being of the child-who-is-a-patient.

Pressured demands and tantrums are common. The outbursts center on "wanting something now" and escalate into threats: "If you don't give me ———— now …" Most unsettling to parents are those statements that culminate in "I'll die if you don't give me ———— now." While children frequently use this expression, its desperation spirals to a searing edge when uttered by an ill child.

Impatience also emerges in more subtle guise, as the wish to hurry the passage of time.

Five-year-old Ricky would only report his age as: "A quarter-to-six which is the same as five-and-a-half." He seemed to be hurrying toward six as if to hasten its arrival. Ricky's advice to Poly Polar Bear on how to get over sadness conveyed the same message: "Play, because playing makes time go faster."

The particular intensity of the life-threatened child reflects his or her existence, dramatically compressed into the present.

Toward the Future

Will I come to see you for the rest of my life? (Jonathan, to the therapist)

References to the future encompass a spectrum from despair, through contingencies of uncertainty, to the hope for certainty. During difficult periods, the only future envisioned by the child is a continuation of the present. Such fatalism can emerge in word or gesture.

Karen wrote a story about being in the hospital that included the startling line: "Every day you wake up to a future of pain."

A hospitalized six-year-old boy just shrugged in response to the therapist's promise to return the next day, as if to say that he placed little stock in "tomorrow."

Ricky, who had just arrived in the clinic after being home for several weeks, informed the therapist: "If I don't feel like talking about dying today, there will be other days."[5] His matter-of-fact plan to talk about endings in the future was devoid of any irony.

The conditional tense lurks behind many of the child's projections into the future. There may not be any particular emphasis on the "if"; the conditional is simply a part of reality.

A ten-year-old girl told the therapist: "If I have a Sweet Sixteen party, I want you to sit at the head table."[6]

Counting on the future is often expressed by a child in whole-hearted optimism and hope. Even when it is based on assumptions that involve a degree of denial, the child's spirit prevails for that time.

We played out the future as children do, as if it were sure to come and as if, when it did, we would be there. It was a game we all played on the ward, even those sure to die.[7]

I like being myself. It is nice being myself. I like being myself forever. (eight-year-old girl)

Although the tenses of time have been examined separately, they are truly inextricable.

A ten-year-old girl stated: "I am afraid that I am going to fall behind in school. Then, when I'm older, I won't know anything." What is evident is her fear in the present, of falling behind into the past, with negative implications for the future.

Karen's book, *My Life Is Feelings,* concludes: "Right now Poly is thinking about the future and what it beholds. Or maybe he is thinking about fun times in the past. He is very happy now as he plays with his train." (See the appendix.)

These examples evoke the stresses and pleasures in the integration of the tenses—the child's synthesis of time.

DREAMS

Ricky: Did you ever have bad dreams?
Therapist: Yes, sometimes I have had bad dreams. Usually when I have bad dreams, it means that I am worried about something.
Ricky: What are your bad dreams, usually?

Therapist: I think that they are a bit like yours. You know, monsters
and things like that.
Ricky: And snakes. . . .
Therapist: What else do you have bad dreams about?
Ricky: A snake biting.
Therapist: When you have those bad dreams, what do you think you
are worrying about?
Ricky: You dying. Everyone dying in the world and leaving me
alone.[8]

The threat of ultimate loss hides, lurks, and emerges in the
dreams of the life-threatened child. The dialogue above culminates
in the revelation of a profound sense of vulnerability. The imagery
of dreams, whether explicit or highly derivative in nature, provides
the child a means of expressing the inexpressible, within the intensity and security of the therapeutic relationship. As Donald Winnicott
wrote: "A dream can be used in therapy since the fact that it *has been
dreamed and remembered and reported* indicates that the material of
the dream is within the capacity of the child, along with the excite-
ments and anxieties that belong to it."[9]

Dream imagery grants the child a degree of separation from the
actuality. In reporting a dream to the therapist, the child can pursue
its connection with current reality to emerge at a new level of disclosure; or, he or she can leave the dream "as is" and experience the relief intrinsic to the process of recounting.

A drawing of a nightmare conveys the ineffable horror that an eleven-
year-old boy was struggling to integrate intrapsychically (color plate
XVII). He portrayed himself in bed, overwhelmed by the image of
a grotesque monster, who is breathing "terror" toward him. The
"terror" resembles traveling cells (metastases?) that are about to invade
the boy's space. Even the colors have a garish, feverish quality. The
word "EEEK," printed in bold letters in the drawing, was the only

verbal accompaniment that the child could offer to describe the dream.

Monsters and devouring animals predominate in the remembered nightmares of the life-threatened child. The oral aggression of the images parallels the invasiveness of the disease process itself. Examples include: "a bear who comes and eats me into little pieces," "alligators coming close to my room," and "sharks eating me." A seven-year-old child who reported nightmares of "a monster after me to take me away," added wistfully that she would rather dream about "a baby duck being feeded." The following interchange with Ricky took place a few weeks after three-year-old Johnny's death:

Ricky reported that he had been having dreams about "monsters, fire-breathing dragons, dinosaurs, and dinosaur rexes." In a counterphobic attempt at control, he bragged: "The next time I have that dream, I'll shoot the monsters with a special gun so that they will melt into ice cubes!" The following day, in a discussion about Johnny, Ricky said: "Johnny is going to come back. I know that he is going to come back, but he will come back different. He will come back as a wild animal." The therapist interpreted: "I wonder if all the dreams you are having about scary wild animals are really your scary thoughts about Johnny's dying." Ricky said: "Yes." In a subsequent session, the therapist asked Ricky if he had slept well the night before. Ricky responded: "Yes. I didn't have any bad dreams. I just had dreams about animals like cats and dogs. TAME—not wild animals." Ricky's nightmares diminished in frequency once the association between the wild animals and Johnny's death was made explicit. Two months later, he reported: "I haven't been having bad dreams. Just thoughts in my head. But I know that they are just in my head." By transforming the unconscious ("bad dreams") into the conscious ("thoughts in my head"), Ricky was exerting a measure of control.

In dreams that involve people, the child often reports similar themes of being chased or devoured.

An eight-year-old girl explained that she slept with her stuffed animals "to protect me from bad people who bite you at night."

Jonathan reported the following dream to his parents. A man is trying to kill him. His sister tries to warn him in time. His parents can't help him. It was this dream, along with his heightened anxiety and obsession with playing "a dying game" that led to his seeing the therapist. A month into the therapy, Jonathan reported a nightmare to the therapist: "A bad lady came up to my sister and me, and said to me: 'You look very tasty.' I asked my sister to pull me back, and I said to that lady: 'No. *You* look very tasty.'" His response to the lady was an attempt at counterattack. The following week, Jonathan drew a storybook in which the themes of his dreams appear (color plates xviii–xxiii). The little mouse in a canoe is being pursued by an aggressive fox (drawn in red, with a sharply angular, wide open mouth). A pale, weak sun is shown in a distant corner of the picture. The fox's parents are waiting for their son to catch the mouse. Two policemen, ordinarily a symbol of active protection to a child of this age, are "just standing around." Like Jonathan's parents in his dream, the policemen seem powerless to help the mouse. At this point, Jonathan became quite agitated and abruptly ended his book with "a monkey swinging." The monkey, although smiling, is suspended precariously between two bare, vulnerable trees—not unlike Jonathan's own life situation. No resolution is offered to the plot of the story; the possibilities were too frightening for him to continue. Regressing to baby talk, Jonathan entitled his book "The Namey-Name Book" and chose stickers of cuddly baby animals to decorate the cover.

"Real-life dreams," stripped of any protective veil, reveal most explicitly the child's life-threatened status. When a child reports such a dream to the parent or therapist, it may simply be a way of notifying the adult of his or her awareness; or, the telling may be an indication of readiness for ongoing discussion.

Karen recounted the following dream to her mother. "I was watching a television show about a busy hectic family. It showed the kids growing up. The youngest child died. It was very sad." The dream was a replication of her own family, in which she was the youngest. Although she declined to discuss the dream further, she had certainly communicated a clear message in its telling. By the time the therapist asked about the dream several days later, Karen claimed to have forgotten it.

A seven-year-old girl had a recurrent dream in the year before her death: "In the dream, I want to be with my mother, and I can never quite get to her." The girl recounted the dream in a joint therapy session with her mother. Whereas the mother found the dream "excruciating," her daughter stipulated that "even though the dream is very sad, it's not a nightmare." The dream provided the focal image for mother and child to work through the anticipatory grief process.[10]

Another theme in the dreams relates to nourishment. Food is a major preoccupation of the seriously ill child, both in reality and in its symbolism of health and nurturance. "Not getting enough" is a reason for worry, if not panic. In the following sequence with Ricky, the issue of "not enough food" expressed through his animals eventually led to the acknowledgment of his mother's worry about him. However, it quickly became evident that to address her concern directly was too threatening. Thus, the therapist, after articulating Ricky's avoidance, accepted it and followed his lead. Ricky returned to the protection afforded by the metaphor of the animals' dreams. The ritualism of each animal's performance—the repetitiveness—is exactly what enabled him to approach the central issue. This is a vivid example of the child's use of dream imagery to work through overwhelming reality.

Ricky had each of the stuffed animals stand up to recount his or her dreams.

Ricky: My wife and sons want to tell their dreams! [as Myrtle
             Dog] "Every night I have a dream that a bigger dog than me

eats up my bone. *That* is serious." And Dacky Raccoon has a problem.

Therapist: What is Dacky's problem?

Ricky: [as Dacky] "Every time I climb up a tree in my dreams, someone always eats my grapes!"

Therapist: It sounds as if nobody gets all the food they are supposed to get!

Ricky: Right—because everyone else eats it.

Therapist: So the animals worry that they are not going to get enough food and nobody will be there to take care of them.

Ricky: [as Quacky Duck] "And I had a dream! Once it was that I had a worm in my refrigerator. SOMEONE ATE IT! ANOTHER DUCK!"

Therapist: Poor Quacky Duck! He didn't get the worm he wanted.

Ricky: [as Poly Polar Bear] "I had a dream once!"

Therapist: Poly Polar Bear is the one who is usually sad.

Ricky: [as Poly Polar Bear] "Yes. I'm sad because once I had a dream that someone ate my fish."

Therapist: Everyone is eating everyone else's food. Nobody is getting enough food.

Ricky: [as Poly Polar Bear, indignantly] "Of course I am getting enough. If someone eats my fish, Daddy will cook me some fried chicken, hamburgers, French fries, potato pancakes, and bean soup."

Therapist: So that means that Daddies take good care of children, even if nobody else does.

Ricky: Uh-huh.

Therapist: Is that true for you, Ricky?

Ricky: Yup.

Therapist: So even though you worry sometimes, you know that your Mommy and Daddy take good care of you.

Ricky: Uh-huh. I think Mommy worries sometimes.

Therapist: You think she worries sometimes? What do you think she worries about?

Ricky:　　　　[to Poly Polar Bear] "I think I know what *your* mother worries about."

Therapist:　What does Poly's mother worry about?

Ricky:　　　　Sometimes she worries that I don't feed Poly enough food. BUT I DO!

Therapist:　That's what Poly's mother worries about. What do you think your mother worries about, Ricky?

Ricky :　　　　[suddenly subdued] I don't know. . . .

Therapist:　Do you think she ever worries?

Ricky:　　　　Do you know, Poly?

Therapist:　[as Poly Polar Bear] "Maybe Ricky's mother worries sometimes . . ." [Ricky begins to make loud animal noises in the background, drowning out the therapist.] Oh, I don't think that Ricky wants to hear about his mother's worries about him. . . .

Ricky:　　　　Look out! Watch out! [He is swinging Poly Polar Bear around as he makes loud noises.]

Therapist:　What's happening to Poly? Poly is falling off the bed and is taking all our attention. I think that is your way of saying that you don't want to talk about your Mommy's worries.

Ricky:　　　　Did all the guys do their dreams yet?

Therapist:　No. How about one more to tell his dreams?

Ricky:　　　　No—a few more. "My name is Spotty Baby Cheetah. I dreamed that SOMEONE EATS MY SEAL."

Therapist:　Someone eats your seal . . . Ricky, all your sons are worried about the same thing.

Ricky:　　　　"My name is Wally Skubeedoo Walrus. And I've got a problem about my dreams. Every time I have a dream, SOME ONE EATS MY FISH."

A few months later, when Ricky was sicker, the theme of "being consumed" appeared in more menacing form in his dreams. Animals were constantly being "pulled into themselves" in a process of self-destruction.

Ricky: I remember I had a dream about a snake that pulled a snake
             into a snake. And then an alligator pulled the alligator into
             the alligator. And a rhino into a rhino into a rhino.
Therapist: All the animals pull themselves into themselves!
Ricky: They eat themselves up!

A related, more horrifying dream image was reported by a dying
eleven-year old girl:

"In my dream, I was nervous and I was chewing my nails. But suddenly I realized that I had chewed up my whole hand. In the dream, I
asked my mother why she didn't stop me, but she didn't answer." This
image of self-consumption (and another example of a parent somehow
unable to protect) was a direct reflection of the girl's own physical state.
She was barely able to eat or drink and thus was literally starving to
death. Her family drawing is a visual analogue to the dream. She
portrayed herself "eating and drinking at the same time at the refrigerator" (figure 31). In the drawing, her hands have disappeared into her
mouth, and she is horizontal, as if she were lying in a coffin.

   Winnicott's affirmation of the child's capacity to deal with a reported dream is always counterbalanced by the therapist's respect for
the child's defenses. When a life-threatened child says, literally or

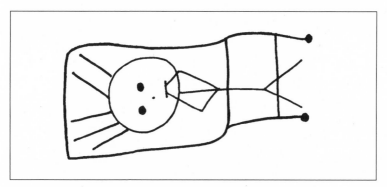

FIGURE 31. *Eating and drinking at the same time*

otherwise, "I can't remember the dream," or "I don't want to talk about it," the therapist must heed the warning. The child may be indicating that reality has overwhelmed the bounds of his or her intrapsychic coping. This is especially true in a child who has been forthcoming about dreams in the past.

At one point, Ricky reported that he had been "sleeping through my dreams." When the therapist pressed him as to what might be scaring him, he answered irritably: "How do I know?" The therapist moved on to more neutral topics.

It is usually the parents who first hear a child's frightening dream. They must soothingly guide the child through and out of the nightmare. However, parents know all too well that the dream reflects the child's immediate reality, not to mention their own. Winnicott writes: "I think it could be said that parents ought not to interpret their children's dreams. The reason for this is that, as is well known, the manifest dream contains an element of defence, and defences must be respected. If one begins to deal with the defenses then one has already turned into a psychotherapist and automatically has moved out of the role of parent."[11]

Even listening to the dreams of their life-threatened child may, at times, exceed the parents' emotional tolerance. Thus, the parents' defenses must also be respected and not overloaded. The distinction between the parents' and the therapist's role in the child's dreamwork is highlighted in the following vignette.

Ricky's mother reported that he had had a bad night. He kept waking his mother to tell her his nightmares. She finally said: "Ricky, I'm tired. I'm not interested in hearing your bad dreams right now." Ricky retorted: "Well, Dr. Sourkes is interested in hearing them."

Frightening dreams are common in a healthy child, so it is not surprising that a seriously ill child may report them more frequently.

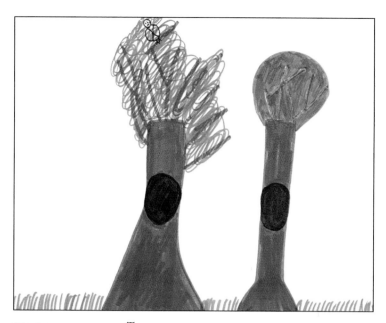

COLOR PLATE XVI. *Trees*

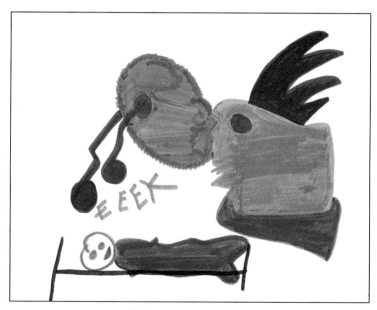

COLOR PLATE XVII. *Nightmare*

The Namey-Name Book

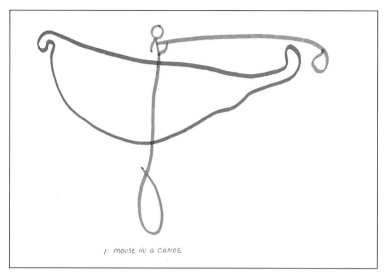

1. mouse in a canoe

COLOR PLATE XVIII.

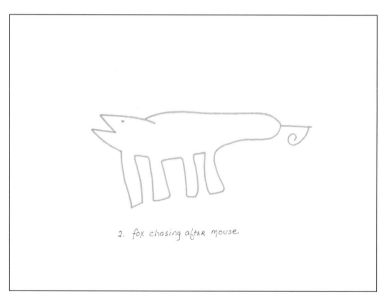

2. fox chasing after mouse

COLOR PLATE XIX.

The Namey-Name Book *(Continued)*

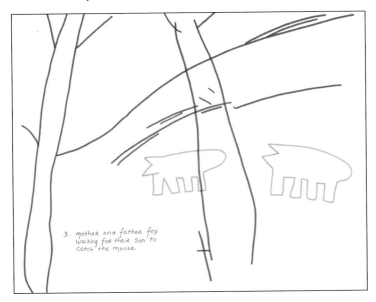

3. mother and father fox
waiting for their son to
catch the mouse

COLOR PLATE XX.

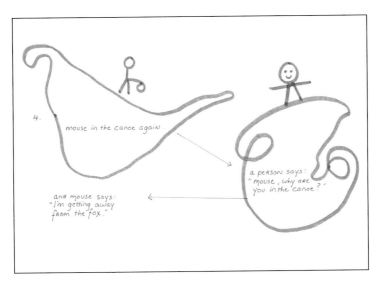

4.

mouse in the canoe again

a person says:
"mouse, why are
you in the canoe?"

and mouse says:
"I'm getting away
from the fox."

COLOR PLATE XXI.

The Namey-Name Book *(continued)*

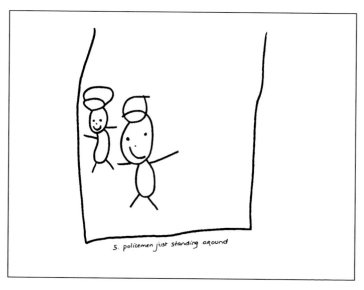

5. policemen just standing around

COLOR PLATE XXII.

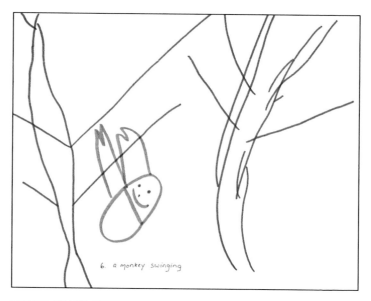

6. a monkey swinging

COLOR PLATE XXIII.

The End

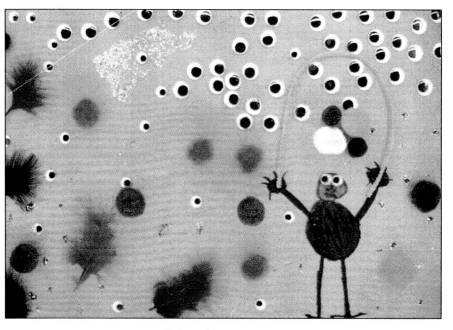

COLOR PLATE XXIV. *God watching over me*

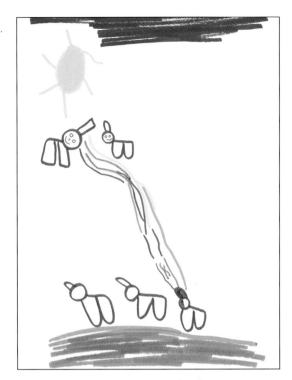

COLOR PLATE XXV. *Unicorn family*

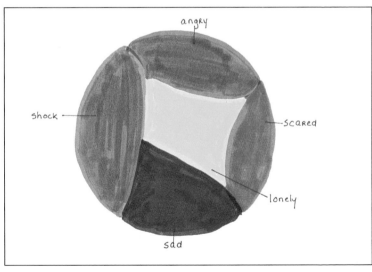

COLOR PLATE XXVI. *How I felt when my friend died*

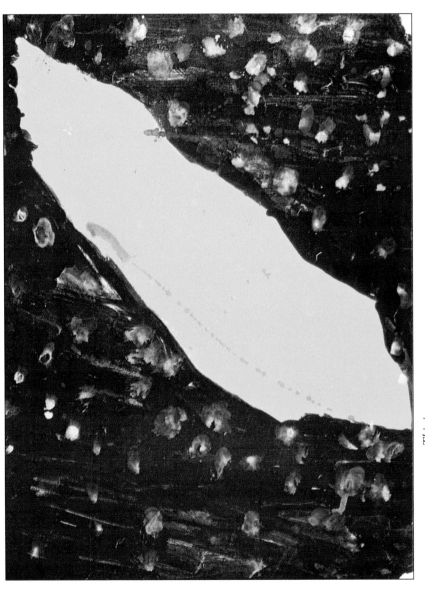

COLOR PLATE XXVII. *This is my space*

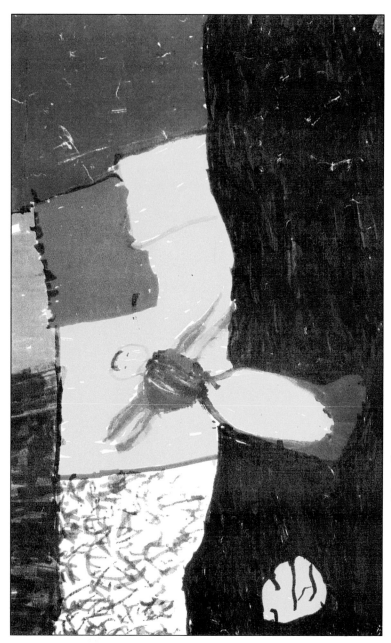

COLOR PLATE XXVIII. *The firefly*

However, a child who has constant nightmares, such that sleep becomes a dreaded time, is clearly overwhelmed by the confluence of intrapsychic and external realities. Through the unconscious communication of the dream, the child is calling out for help in managing what feels unmanageable. As the terror is brought to light in psychotherapy, the intensity and frequency of the nightmares diminish.

SPIRITUALITY

To live is to love. (Karen)

I kept thinking [my son's] time in the children's ward would irrevocably change him. A shadow was falling across his vision of life.[12]

The child who has been diagnosed with a life-threatening illness can be quite pensive about the meaning of life and death. His or her view of the world reflects a precocious awareness of the fragility of life. While "spirituality" certainly includes religion, it encompasses broader existential concerns. The child tries to make sense of what has happened in order to put his or her individual situation into a broader context. Robert Coles says that in circumstances of serious illness, "psychological themes connect almost imperceptibly, but quite vividly at moments, with a spiritual inwardness."[13] The child's reflections on life are framed by that struggle toward survival.

> Life is so strange. Sometimes you feel it's like a
> book with chapters to fill, never ending.
> Sometimes it's like a chess game where you have
> to make each move so carefully.
> Other times it's like a mystery where each hidden
> chamber reveals its secrets.
> It is even a war, where to live it is to win it.[14]
> (Karen)

At times, such views may border on the cynical. Innocence has been shattered, and nothing is taken for granted.

A ten-year-old boy whose parents were going through a divorce, said: "I wonder sometimes what I fought for. The leukemia, the leukemia again, the transplant, and now the separation ... Is this what it all comes to? I thought that after the transplant, we would be one big happy family, but life isn't always what you want." Karen expressed similar sentiments in describing a friend: "Maybe she expects too much out of life."

The therapist must be open to exploring concerns at the confluence of the psychological and the spiritual. Often the essence of what the child is struggling to understand lies within that uncharted territory.

In the days following Johnny's death, Ricky asked: "What does 'spirit' mean? Nobody knows all the answers, right?" The therapist encouraged Ricky to talk about all the things that he remembered about Johnny, including what he looked like, the games he enjoyed, what made him laugh. After reminiscing, the therapist concluded that the "spirit" of Johnny was in all these memories that Ricky could hold. Ricky seemed satisfied with this explanation.

Issues of faith—and loss of faith—arise even in the very young child. It is common for a child in a religious family to find comfort in those beliefs. His or her observance may intensify, whether through attending services or through more frequent prayers and discussions at home. Whereas some children's sense of trust may be shaken ("How could God let this happen to me?"), most perceive God as their savior in the battle with the illness.

An eight-year-old boy had gone to the doctor to check his injuries after falling down the stairs. Through this examination and subsequent blood tests, he had been diagnosed with leukemia. The boy explained:

"God made me fall down the stairs so that the doctors would find the disease in my body and treat it."

Karen advised Poly Polar Bear to pray to God for help with his problems: "If you don't know any prayers from books, then make up your own. They *sometimes* [italics added] work." She then wrote an example for him:

> The Lord almighty
> with his great power and wisdom
> Can see farther than the human eye.
> So if he now watches over me
> Just let me be nice and healthy.

In the following two drawings, one child invests in God's omnipresent protection, while the other comments on God's passivity.

An eight-year-old boy who has just relapsed worked on his picture in the playroom. In response to the child life specialist's query about all the "eyes" that he had so carefully glued onto the paper, he explained: "It's God watching over me" (color plate xxiv).[15]

A five-year-old girl drew each member of her family engaged in an activity and included a figure without arms and legs whom she labeled "God." She stated matter-of-factly: "God is a part of our family, every family. He's not doing anything" (figure 32).

When the child has a question related to his or her own religion, it is often prudent to encourage discussion of the issue with the parents or a member of the clergy. This is especially true when the child has already been given partial information or when the queries are persistent. The therapist must take the utmost care not to intrude on the family's belief system, either through ignorance or contradictory ideas.

The following interchange with Ricky took place about two

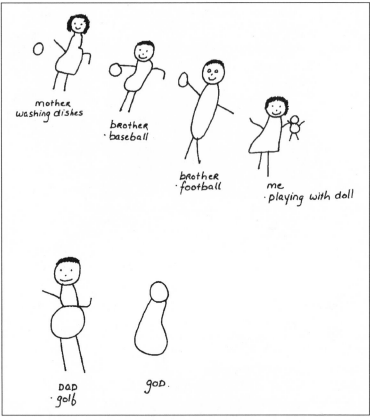

FIGURE 32. *Family: God is a part of our family*

weeks after his questions about "spirit." When the therapist asked Ricky whether he wanted to talk about going home (scheduled for later that week) or about his dreams, he replied: "I'd like to talk about dying."

Therapist: What are you thinking about, Ricky? What are you interested in about dying?

Ricky: About how do they come down? Daddy says that when peo-

ple die, God decides when they should stay up there or
when they should come down.

Therapist: I don't really know about those things. That's something
that you should ask Daddy more about.

Ricky: He says that when people go up to heaven, God decides
when they should be up there for a long time, or when they
should come down here.

Therapist: I think that you're going to have to ask Daddy about that,
because I really don't know. Do you promise to ask him?

Ricky: All right. Let's talk about the food that Grandma makes for
me. . . .

The child may seek to imbue death with new meaning. Even if
the child holds a traditional religious view of the afterlife, he or she
may attempt to reframe death in a way that grants a form of continuity, or provides a cosmic context for its occurrence.

Karen reinterpreted Saint-Exupéry's *The Little Prince* in the following
way: "It's not that sad because he didn't really die—he just went back to
his own planet." It was during this period that she developed an interest in reincarnation: "Death is like sleep, and I'm half not afraid because I believe in reincarnation."

Amy wrote this poem and set it to music:

> Someday as we are all quiet
> the sun will stop
> shining and the world
> will stop. All that will
> be heard is music.

Spirituality is a wellspring, an inner belief system or resource
from which the child can draw strength and solace. The therapist
who is conscious of this dimension enables the child to express his
or her hopes, loves, and values in the struggle to live. Whether

framed in terms of humanism, nature, or religion, spirituality contributes to the child's ego-strength and resilience in coping with extraordinary stress.

The child's awareness of mortality emerges in different forms throughout the course of the illness. Allusions to time, and reflections about dreams and spirituality illuminate the intrapsychic underpinnings of the experience. Inextricably linked to the horizons of awareness is the process of anticipatory grief: the threat of loss extends to encompass the child in relationship to others.

✤ Anticipatory Grief

Therapist: What does it mean to be alive?
Ricky: That your family doesn't miss you. They miss you if
            you die. When you're alive, you don't miss people
            because they are right here.[1]

Loss, as the core of anticipatory grief, can be conceptualized along three intersecting axes: loss of control, loss of identity, and loss of relationships.[2] While loss of control extends over emotional issues, and ultimately over life itself, its emergence is most vivid in the child's day-to-day experience of the illness, in the barrage of intrusive, uncomfortable, or painful procedures that he or she must endure. The child strives desperately to regain a measure of control, often expressed through resistant, noncompliant behavior or aggressive outbursts. Too often, the source of the anger—the loss of control—goes unrecognized by parents and caregivers. However, once its meaning is acknowledged, an explicit distinction may be drawn for the child between what he or she can or cannot dictate. In order to maximize the child's sense of control, the environment can be structured to allow for as much choice as is feasible. Even options that appear small or inconsequential serve as an antidote to loss, and their impact is often reflected in dramatic improvements in behavior.

Issues surrounding loss of identity are not pronounced in the young child for the simple reason that identity formation is a developmental task of adolescence.[3] However, the child does grapple with self-recognition. The distinction between before and after, same and different (relative to self and to others), normal and abnormal, are all facets of the child's struggle to maintain a constant sense of self and not to lose him or herself to the illness.

Loss of relationships—expressed through fears of separation, absence, and death—is paramount in anticipatory grief: "grief expressed in advance when the loss is perceived as inevitable."[4] A broader definition includes loss that is felt to be threatening or lurking around the edges of awareness, even if not inevitable. Anticipatory grief may show itself as the child's increased sensitivity to separation, without any specific reference to death; comments or questions related to death that may be seen as a type of preparation or rehearsal; and the undiluted and unmistakable grief of the terminal phase of the illness. Thus, while anticipatory grief is catapulted into being at the time of diagnosis, its manifestation throughout the illness trajectory will differ depending upon whether the child is living with a life-threatening diagnosis, but doing well; the child is going to die, but not imminently; or the child is actually dying.

Undergirding the child's fear of separation in daily life is a powerful sense of *separateness,* of being apart, regardless of others' supportive presence. Quite often, the child omits him or herself from a family drawing, even when the instruction to "draw *everyone* in your family" has been emphasized. In a psychiatric population, leaving oneself out of a family drawing suggests psychopathology or dysfunction in the child or the family system. However, in life-threatening illness, the hesitation to draw oneself, or an outright omission, more often reflects the reality of the child's situation. In other versions of being apart, the child may portray him or herself "en-

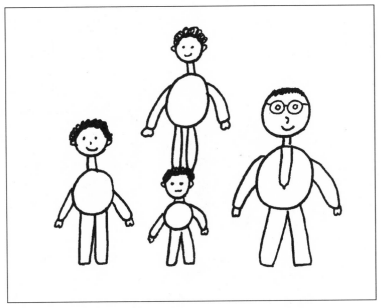

FIGURE 33. *Family: I forgot myself*

closed" or distant from the rest of the family, often with intimations of death.

When Jonathan was asked to do a family drawing, he asked the therapist matter-of-factly: "Do I have to make me?" He then complied willingly, although he drew himself last.

A seven-year-old girl cheerfully announced that she had finished her picture, after having methodically drawn her parents and younger brother. When the therapist casually asked: "And what about you?" she responded, startled: "Oh! I forgot!" Only then did the girl put herself into the picture—solidly on top of her brother's head (figure 33). This triumphant placement reflected the resentment that she had been expressing to her mother in recent weeks: "Why is he always so healthy and I'm so sick all the time?" [5]

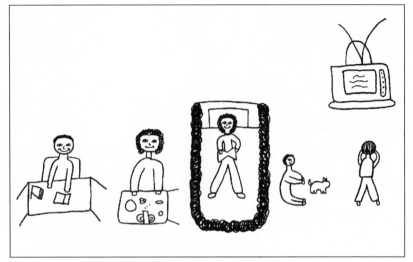

FIGURE 34. *Family: Reading in bed*

In a family portrait, a ten-year-old girl depicted herself as "reading in bed." Her passive posture within the starkly ruffled bed connotes an open coffin (figure 34).

Soon after his diagnosis, a five-year-old boy drew a picture of a family of unicorns (color plate xxv). He explained that it was a mother, father, and sister unicorn on the ground, and a brother unicorn up in the sky with God. Although he did not further identify the unicorns, or specify which two are linked by the rainbow, he did replicate his own family constellation. Only the brother and God are smiling, as if they are more "alive" than the faceless unicorns on the ground. There had been no discussion of death with this child, nor had he known any children who had died.[6]

Themes of presence and absence, disappearance and return, may be evident in the child's play, both in psychotherapy sessions and at home. Elaborate versions of hide-and-seek actually mirror the concerns of "not being here," the crux of anticipatory grief. The child is also testing whether his or her absence would be noticed and whether he or she would be missed.

Jonathan proposed a game to the therapist: "When I snap my fingers, I'll disappear." He would hide somewhere in the office with several small toy animals. While Jonathan was "invisible" to the therapist, she would do a monologue wondering where he could be, progressing from innocuous to more threatening possibilities: "I wonder whether Jonathan is in school and that's why I can't find him.... Maybe he went down to the cafeteria.... Maybe he's not feeling well.... I wonder whether something happened to Jonathan.... I would be sad if something happened to him.... Everyone would miss him...." Jonathan would listen intently to her words, without answering. At a certain point he would throw a small animal out of his hiding place for the therapist to question about his whereabouts. Eventually, one of the animals, through the therapist's voice, would "tell" where Jonathan was hiding. He would reappear with a bound, and the therapist would greet him with enthusiasm and relief. Jonathan played this ritual over many sessions.

The child may express frequent or intense missing of close friends and relatives whom he or she does not often see. Hospitalization, in particular, provokes talk about missing certain people. Such longing is predicated on attachment and thus is inextricable with the experience of loss.

The child's fear of missing his or her caregivers arises most often toward the end of an extended hospitalization, when the contact has been intense, or when there are long breaks between scheduled clinic appointments. The child admits honestly that "I won't miss getting my medicines, but I will miss seeing you." If he or she lives far from the treatment center, the sense of geographical distance intensifies the reaction. While the separation from the caregivers is usually positive, in that the child is returning to his or her "outside" life, recognition of the anticipatory missing is crucial preparation for the leave-taking.

Ricky was being discharged home for a month's break between courses of treatment. He told the therapist that he was "a little bit scared" of going home and leaving the therapist "alone." What then emerged was his fear of missing the therapist:

Therapist: I am going to miss you too. I wonder what it will be like to miss each other....
Ricky: [shakes his head]
Therapist: You are shaking your head.... I don't know what that means.
Ricky: [whispering] That means no.
Therapist: That means no? That means ...
Ricky: That means it wouldn't be too good to miss each other.[7]

In another manifestation of anticipatory grief, the child projects concern about him or herself onto a significant adult, usually a parent or the therapist. On one level, the child recognizes his or her extreme dependence on the adult and panics at the thought of something happening to that person. This reaction may be particularly pronounced in the child of a single parent. On another level, the child is expressing fear about his or her own situation through this mirror image. At least initially, the projection is best left untouched, as the child is clearly communicating extreme vulnerability.

A nine-year-old girl repeatedly asked her mother: "What would happen to me if something happened to you?"

After a discussion about his bad dreams, the therapist asked Ricky what else he felt scared about.

Ricky: I am scared of what if my mother dies. Then there will be no one to take care of me.

Therapist: I know that your mother takes good care of herself and is healthy so that she can take good care of you.

Ricky: Yes. She is trying very hard to stay alive. She eats all the time and she kisses me a lot.

Therapist: What else are you scared about?

Ricky: I am scared that when I come back to the hospital, you will not be here.

The child's grief related to the possibility of his or her own dying may be cloaked in symbolic terms or in questions about others. As in all other communications, the therapist must stay close to the immediate concern, leaving the child in control of how far to pursue the topic. Often he or she will make an isolated statement, or pose one question, and then, without further comment, turn to other subjects. It is as if the child is "gathering data" and knows just how much he or she can absorb at a given time. Parents will often comment that they have been taken aback, even stunned, by the unexpected nature of these disclosures.

A three-year-old boy was walking through the woods with his parents during the autumn. When his father explained that the leaves change color and then fall off the trees, the boy burst into tears: "I don't like those trees. They're dead." The following spring, the parents described his "grief" (their word) over a tree that didn't produce leaves.

Ricky asked his mother how old people are when they die. When she responded that people usually die when they are very old, he commented that he didn't want his grandmother to die. A few days later, he asked about an uncle who had died when Ricky was only a year old and whom he had never mentioned before.

The most powerful disclosures are those in which the child makes reference to the possibility of his or her own dying. Whether through the weight of the sadness or through the actual words or images, there is no doubt that the child is grieving. Such evidence of the anticipatory grief process emerges at every point in the illness trajectory, even in the child who goes on to be cured.

Ricky animatedly told the therapist: "Wally Skubeedoo Walrus's birthday is November fourteenth." The therapist asked Ricky the date of *his* birthday. He answered: "November fourteenth. All my sons and daughters are on November fourteenth. Too bad you're not also." The therapist then asked him how old he would be on November fourteenth. Ricky's affect changed markedly, and he responded very quietly: "Six...." Ricky's excited anticipation collapsed into sadness when the birthday was personalized to his own growing up into the future.

Jonathan came into a session in good spirits, although somewhat subdued. He reported that his teacher and friends had been happy to see him on his return to school. When the therapist asked whether Jonathan had been happy to see them, he did not answer. His silence conveyed sadness, a recognition of being apart from the rest of the class. The quality of the silence was much like Ricky's response to thinking about his birthday.

A four-year-old boy inquired of his mother: "Will you cry when I die?" His question was matter-of-fact, and he listened intently as his mother explained that she *would* cry if he died, but that he was doing well on treatment, and so she was sure that he wouldn't die until he was very old. She thus addressed the emotional component of the question honestly, while adding reassurance.

Upon hearing that she had relapsed, a ten-year-old girl informed her parents of where she wanted to be buried and asked whom she "had" in heaven.

Past losses loom large for the child who has been diagnosed with a life-threatening illness. Grief that had previously been resolved may have to be reworked in light of current experience. Some children report a strong sense of connection to the person who died; the identification seems to provide a certain measure of protection or comfort. Pets who have died are also invoked with intensity.

Jenny had lost her father (through illness) and her best friend (in an accident) in the three years prior to her own diagnosis. She always brought a stuffed animal that her father had given her into the hospital and spoke frequently about her best friend.

Just before a seven-year-old girl got sick, her mother had given birth to a stillborn boy. The girl talked obsessively about him to the therapist: "When I die, I'll see him. But I'm not planning to die. But I want to see my brother, my dog, and my grandpa. My grandpa died before I was born. I still think about my brother. If he hadn't died, he'd be the littlest. I feel bad when I think about him. I wish he were alive."

An eight-year-old girl chattered incessantly about her two guinea pigs who had died before she got sick: "The first guinea pig died—he CROAKED! He was only a baby, but he was the runt of the family. They always die first. I was sad, but it was even worse when the second one died."

Deaths that occur while the child is being treated provoke intense anxiety and sadness. Developmentally appropriate concerns and questions about death are amplified by the child's own situation.

A four-year-old boy's grandfather had died a few weeks prior to the session. His anxiety was palpable as he began to talk: "My grandpa died. He looked different when he was dead. He's still dead. My grandpa was sick. He was in a lot of pain and suffering." By bringing Kiss the Squirrel into the discussion, the therapist provided the boy "company" in his loss and opened a parallel avenue for disclosure.

Therapist: Kiss was sad because he missed you. His grandfather
            died too.

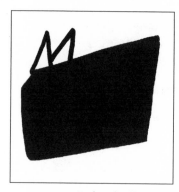

FIGURE 35. *Bed and pillow*

Child: Is his grandfather still dead? Which grave is he in?

Therapist: Yes, his grandfather is still dead. He is in a grave near the nut trees.

Child: My grandfather's grave is in our town.

After this interchange, the boy drew a solid black bed and pillow (figure 35), its ominous quality reminiscent of a grave. He then proceeded "to give chemo" to Kiss. At the end of the hour, he and the therapist reviewed the session:

Therapist: We did a lot of things today. We gave Kiss his chemo . . . we talked about sad things . . . your grandfather . . .

Child: And Kiss's grandfather! I'm going to tell Mommy.

An elderly neighbor of a ten-year-old girl died. The woman had been a surrogate grandmother through the child's years of illness and treatment. The girl attended the funeral—her first. That night, she dreamed that she went to visit the woman (now a ghost), who was sitting with other ghosts at her kitchen table. The girl was scared and tried to run away from the woman-ghost who began to chase her. After recounting the dream, she picked up a cuddly animal puppet, and began to speak in baby talk. Her regression—the first time ever in a session—was a direct response to the overwhelming anxiety of the day and to the image of being chased by death.

The death of another patient engenders an inextricable combination of grief and anticipatory grief and spirals the child into a peak of vulnerability. Thoughts about separation, dying, and death, usually relegated to the background, surge forward into consciousness. Although the heightened anticipatory grief abates within hours, days, or weeks, profound sadness endures. The child's view of his or her own illness is irrevocably changed by the evidence that the possibility of death can be transformed into actuality. This is especially true of the first death that the child encounters. Multiple losses, not uncommon in the child's experience over time, are ongoing intimations of mortality.

It is best that the child be gently informed of another patient's death by the parents or a close caregiver. However difficult it is to relay the news, undue delay or avoidance heighten the risk of the child finding out "accidentally," without the benefit of the adult's protective presence. Certainly some unexpected disclosures do occur, especially for a child who comes into the medical center infrequently. Thus, the child may ask casually about another patient, only to find out that he or she has died; or someone may refer to this patient, assuming that the child already knew. Whether the child learns of the death while in the hospital or at home, the parents and caregivers must be attuned and available. The following vignettes illustrate the gamut of reactions—sadness, fear, and anger—unleashed by the death of another patient.

In the first child's conversation with his mother and the therapist, he quickly focused on the separation from parents—a core concern. His later flight from the deceased child's parents highlights the fear of "death by association."

A five-year-old boy heard about another patient's death on a visit to the clinic. A discussion ensued with his mother and the therapist:

Child: Susie died.
Therapist: How did she die?
Child: 'Kemia. I'm going to miss her. I wish she'd come back.
Mother: Susie's with God now. She's happy.
Child: Are her mommy and daddy with her?

A few months later, at the clinic's Christmas party, the boy ran away when he caught sight of Susie's parents.

Many critical issues are highlighted in the next selection. A child's response to the news of another's death often takes time to emerge. Initially he or she may be too overwhelmed to say or do anything. Furthermore, sensing the parents' grief, the child may try to protect them from witnessing his or her anguish. In a common defensive maneuver, the child differentiates—and thus distances—his or her own medical status from that of the patient who has died. This is not the juncture for the adult to debate the "truth" of such evaluations; tacit agreement, if not outright reassurance, is usually in order. Given the episodic nature of the expression of grief in childhood (in contrast to the continuity of the underlying feelings), the therapist should periodically invoke the name of the dead child, to prevent unmentioned grief from becoming unmentionable.

Ricky did not say very much when his mother informed him of Johnny's death. However, when his physician walked into the room a few hours later, Ricky pointed to the ceiling, asking: "Where is he up there? Where did he go? My medicines work!" At the end of the day, the therapist came in.

Therapist: I hear you got some sad news today.
Ricky: Yah.
Therapist: That Johnny died.... How did you feel?
Ricky: Scared.
Therapist: Scared about what?
Ricky: That he's up there.... How did he die? Did they lose control?

It was at this juncture that the therapist introduced the alive-dead game for the first time. After playing it, Ricky sat back and looked at his stuffed animals assembled around the bed.

Therapist: Ricky, look at Poly Polar Bear. He looks very sad and is not playing.

Ricky: Is he sad because Johnny died?

Therapist: I guess so. What shall we do?

Ricky: Play!

Therapist: You mean that when you play, you don't feel so sad about Johnny?

Ricky: Yes!

In a session a few days later, the therapist picked up Poly Polar Bear and commented that he still looked sad. Without any hesitation, Ricky asked: "Do you think that he is still sad because Johnny died?" The next day, all the animals, including Poly Polar Bear, were angry and fighting when the therapist walked in. When she asked what Poly was mad about, Ricky said: "Maybe because Johnny died." A week later, Ricky commented that Poly was "sad all over again about Johnny." He picked up Poly and said to him: "Well, all Johnny's medicines didn't work and they lost control and that's all.... I'm glad my medicines work." The therapist then did a monologue about Poly being afraid of what would happen if he got sick and his medicines didn't work. Ricky listened intently. When the therapist brought in the tape recorder the following week, she "interviewed" Ricky about his experiences:

Therapist: What happened here about a friend of yours a few weeks ago that was very sad?

Ricky: [interrupting] Who? Johnny?

Therapist: Could you tell people about what happened to Johnny? What did it feel like for you?

Ricky: Mommy told me.

Therapist: Mommy told you. Why don't you tell people, because they don't know about Johnny.

Ricky: All right. JOHNNY DIED AND HE WENT UP TO HEAVEN.

Therapist: How did he die, Ricky?

Ricky: They ran out of medicine. And when they ran out of medicine, he just died. His heart stopped beating. They lost control.

Therapist: They lost control of his illness, right?

Ricky: Uh-huh. His was bigger than mine, I think.

Therapist: Sounds like his was bigger than yours. And how did you feel when your mommy told you that Johnny had died?

Ricky: Not too good. And then you came in. And I played.

Therapist: Can you tell me a little more about how you felt?

Ricky: [in a wail] Sad that I missed Johnny.

Therapist: And then I came in and we talked and played, and what started to happen?

Ricky: I started to feel better!

In the last example, the child provides a synthesis of the reactions to the death of another patient. In having the same illness, an extra layer of identification infuses the experience.

Through a mandala (color plate XXVI), an eleven-year-old girl described her reaction to the death of her friend. Both had leukemia and had known each other since the age of six. "I knew he was sick, but not *that* sick [*shock*—green]. One minute he was about to have a bone marrow transplant—the next minute he was dead. I was so *sad* [blue] because he died. I was *angry* [purple] that it happened to him, that he died on his birthday. The nurses were going to have a party for him—it was awful. He should have died after his birthday, so he could have died happy, or happier. I was *afraid* [red] that it might happen to me. I've heard about a lot of kids who have died. I have a book that says you can die from leukemia. I felt *lonely* [yellow] because he's the only one I really knew at the clinic. I looked forward to seeing him. Now when we visit his family, his little brother reminds me of him." After the child had completed her mandala, she added: "I asked my parents if I could go to my friend's wake. At first they said no. But I reminded them that he was more my friend than theirs, so they let me go." In the following session, she reported having felt "sad for the rest of the day" after talking about her friend.

The Fear of Replacement

The fear of being replaced looms for the child and may find expression either directly or through play. To replace makes explicit the fact that something has been lost or has ceased to exist. Thus, for the child, replacement carries with it the recognition of his or her own mortality. Some children may manifest this fear through an upsurge in resentment toward a younger sibling perceived as being in line to take his or her place. In another vein, the child may be extremely sensitive to any attachments the parents develop toward children other than their own. Most complicated are the intensely ambivalent feelings that arise if the mother becomes pregnant while the child is still in active treatment. Obviously he or she fears losing the parents' attention and availability. Often not articulated, however, is the child's suspicion that the parents are having another child as an insurance policy against his or her death. In some instances, the child has accurately read the parents' motivation. More frequently, however, despite the hardship of the child's illness, the parents are simply proceeding with their family's development as they had previously envisioned it.

One day, to Karen's chagrin, she found that a stuffed dog had been added to the therapist's toy collection. She named him Droopy (because of his droopy ears). Karen spent the session having Poly Polar Bear beat up Droopy, while discussing with Poly the advantages and disadvantages of having a younger brother. In the subsequent session, the following exchange ensued:

Karen: Droopy's okay, I guess, but I still like Poly Polar Bear better. I wonder why Poly doesn't like Droopy at all.

Therapist: Maybe he's jealous that we might like Droopy too much. But Poly should know that he is special. . . .

Karen: And NOBODY can take his place.[8]

The therapist simultaneously highlighted the issue of replacement while assuring Karen (through Poly) of her own special place.

An eight-year-old girl saw a school photograph of the daughter of a family friend in her father's wallet. This picture was in addition to many of his own children. The child exploded in rage, accusing her father of not loving her any more since he carried a photograph of another girl.

A four-year-old girl's discharge from a long hospitalization was contingent on her beginning to eat adequately. Her mother was eight months pregnant at the time. The therapist suggested that the staff encourage the child to eat without articulating the explicit goal of going home, since "home" meant facing the imminent arrival of the new baby. Once the connection was broken, the girl gradually began to eat.

A less common, but more salutary interpretation of replacement may emerge when a child hears of another's death. He or she suggests that the parents have another child to replace the one who has died in order to restore normalcy and fill the loss. Embedded may be the magical thought that the "replacement" will in fact be the "return" of the one who died, thus assuaging the child's own fear of death. This view of the replacement child as a comfort, rather than as a threat, often goes unrecognized by the therapist.

One of Ricky's initial comments after Johnny's death was: "I told my parents that Johnny's parents should have another Johnny." He seemed to present the idea as an immediate solution to the loss. When the therapist explained to Ricky that each child is different and unique, and that one child cannot substitute for another, Ricky listened quietly and then, without any further comment said: "Let's play." The therapist's explanation had been offered in the belief that "being irreplaceable" would be of comfort to Ricky, not realizing that his vision was of Johnny being replaced by the very same Johnny. Ricky's subdued reaction, and change of subject indicated that the therapist had inadvertently taken away some of his own hope for himself.

A child's tenacity in holding on to his or her own belief system, even in the face of contradictory ideas presented by the therapist, is impressive.

In completely different terms from the above conversation about Johnny, but with the same theme, Ricky reported the following dream a few weeks later:

Ricky: A friendly snake and a friendly worm found an alligator. The alligator wanted to shoot the worm, so the snake shot the alligator instead.

Therapist: What happened to the alligator?

Ricky: He died. The ice came. The ice ages came.

Therapist: And was it sad in your dream when he died?

Ricky: Of course it was. His friends missed him. But his nephew grew up and looked just like the alligator. So the alligator's friends didn't know which one was which!

By this time it was evident to the therapist that Ricky's belief in replacement was an antidote to his fear of death, and thus should be left intact.

The child's fear of replacement cannot be eliminated entirely, although it certainly can be worked through in psychotherapy and assuaged by the parents' reassurance. A preoccupation with being replaced usually signifies the child's need to talk about his or her life-threatening situation, with particular focus on the fear of death. In addition, the child is often speaking for the family's difficulty in negotiating the possibility of loss.

Therapist: Are you in any pain? Does anything hurt?

Jenny: My heart.

Therapist: Your heart?
Jenny: My heart is broken.... I miss everybody.[9]

The distillation of anticipatory grief to its essence marks the imminence of death. At times imperceptibly, at other times dramatically, the child who has been living with the illness is transformed into a dying child.

✤ The Dying Child

Reach out and take it, little girl,
It will be here sooner than you think.
Reach out and tell them, little girl,
You'll be on your way soon.
Don't cry now 'cause it's your day.
It's here already, see?

(Amy)

The dying child faces the ultimate leave-taking, the departure from all that is familiar and loved. There are two phases in the dying process. In a broad sense, the child is in the terminal phase when the illness no longer responds to conventional treatment. The emphasis of therapy shifts from a curative approach to palliative care. Yet the child may continue to live quite productively for weeks or months, either on experimental treatment or on no treatment at all. In a more delimited sense, *terminal* refers to the endpoint, when, regardless of the status of treatment, death is imminent. However the term is used, physical and psychological comfort are of utmost importance during the terminal phase. Even when treatment continues with the goal of prolonging life for a brief period, its major emphasis is on symptom control and support.[1]

Throughout the terminal phase, the child is often aware of the diminishing, or nonexistent, options that he or she faces. It is at this time that the child may ask anxiously: "What if this medicine doesn't work? What will you give me next?" The child experiences a profound sense of loss of control.

In the last year of her life, Karen's parents kept a list of available research drugs. Karen would occasionally comment with relief: "I still have [for example] three to go."

An eleven-year-old child explained: "One side of my head says: 'Think optimistic.' The other side says: 'What if this treatment doesn't work?'"

Decisions during the terminal phase are difficult, since there can no longer be any promise of prolonged time. The parents do not want their child to suffer more, yet they often cannot tolerate the thought of ending treatment, of "leaving any stone unturned." The role of the physician and the caregiving team shifts from leadership in recommending a treatment plan to the clarification of remaining options and consequences. The choice between experimental treatment versus cessation usually revolves around the child's quality of life and the family's comfort with the idea of terminating treatment. In most instances, the parents make the decision; however, to varying degrees, the child may be involved in such discussions.

A seven-year-old girl told her parents that she was too tired to fight any more and that she wanted to give up. She added: "If I have to continue suffering, I would rather be in heaven." These statements were major determinants in the parents' choosing a palliative care plan without any further treatment for her.

An eleven-year-old girl was offered the option of radiation therapy for pain control. She said: "I'm scared because I'm not so good at making decisions. My parents want me to have radiation, but a little voice in me tells me not to. . . . My mother always said that if I die, she wants me to die happy and at home. If I had radiation, I'd have to come into the hospital every day. And I don't know if radiation will really help, or if I would die anyway."

During the terminal phase, the child's awareness of dying becomes more focused. No longer an abstract threat in the distance, death takes on an identity of its own. Rather than being a possible outcome, death is *the* outcome, its time of occurrence the only unknown. References to its proximity can be quite direct and explicit. If an open climate has been established from the beginning of the illness, it will be reflected in how the child talks about death.

An eleven-year-old girl commented: "Some of my friends have died. I wish I could talk to those kids' parents to see what their symptoms were, so that I would know what is happening to me."

A few months before his death, an eight-year-old boy called out from the bedroom to his parents: "Am I dying?"

The awareness may also be expressed symbolically, although no less powerfully, through play and art.

A four-year-old boy incorporated "dead" into much of his play in the weeks before his death. For example, he rolled back the plastic eyes of one of his stuffed animals, so that they looked closed, and informed the therapist: "He's dead." After a brief silence, he added quickly: "But they made him okay now." The boy then turned over as if to sleep. A few minutes later, he said: "My teddy bear was all curled up and they put him away."

A three-year-old boy played the same game with a stuffed duck and a toy ambulance each time he was hospitalized. The duck would be sick and need to go to the hospital by ambulance. The boy would move the ambulance, making siren noises.

Therapist: How is the duck?
Child: Sick.
Therapist: Where is he going?
Child: To the hospital.

Therapist: What are they going to do?
Child: Make him better.
Therapist: Is he going to get better?
Child: Yes, better.

During what turned out to be the boy's terminal admission, he played the same game with the duck. However, the ritual changed dramatically in its outcome:

Therapist: How is the duck?
Child: Sick.
Therapist: Is he going to get better?
Child: [shaking his head slowly] Ducky not get better. Ducky die.[2]

In the weeks before his death, a boy did a series of drawings around the themes of space and light (color plate xxvii). He described a yellow shaft of light headed into the dark beyond as: "Space. This is space. This is my space." Two days later, he drew a vibrant firefly, smiling broadly as it emerges from the blackness into the central light (color plate xxviii). He said: "Fireflies glow in the dark and show others the way." This was his last picture or activity; he went to bed that evening and never came downstairs again.

Catastrophic images often emerge in the child's language and stories during the terminal phase. Fear, desperation, and the sense of disaster are all evident, even if in derivative form.

A four-year-old boy in the intensive care unit focused on a stretcher outside his room: "See the bed out there? It's a dead bed." He then began to chant: "Dead bed, code red, they call you that when you're dead."

Ricky recounted the following story to the therapist in the months before his death: "The TV fell off the wall and the IV pole crashed on the dinosaur and then the lights turned out and then the bed turned back to the wall. The door slammed, the walls fell, and the hospital broke down on the dinosaur."[3]

Some parents, recognizing the hopelessness of their own child's situation, demonstrate an intensified interest in another patient, particularly one who is "doing well." This is a manifestation of anticipatory grief gone awry and causes inordinate suffering. In the eyes of the child, being replaced by another patient is the ultimate betrayal. Furthermore, the child feels that in "failing" the treatment, he or she has failed the parents, and thus the replacement is perceived as punishment.

As the child confronts impending death, he or she may show signs of preparation. The child's actions or words are often quite matter-of-fact; their significance is not necessarily elaborated.

In the last months of her life, a seven-year-old girl gave many of her favorite possessions to family members and friends. She had several conversations with her parents about death and about wanting to be buried with her grandfather. The girl mused that she would be able to tell a deceased friend that she had recently seen his mother.

A few months before her death, Karen said to her mother: "You know which toys I want to go with me. You know what I mean, so don't make me say it."

The dying child's anticipatory grief is palpable, as he or she lives the intensity of separation in its ultimate form. Sadness permeates many departures.

A five-year-old boy would ordinarily wave good-bye to everyone as a group at family gatherings. On this occasion, he went around the room and kissed each person individually. The next week, the boy repeated the ritual with each nurse in the clinic. In both situations, it was as if he knew that this might be his last good-bye.

Jonathan said: "Good-bye, house" as his parents drove him to the hospital for what became his terminal admission.

The parents need information about how the child is likely to die, and, in some instances, support in coming to a decision about a home or hospital death. Effective pain control is a critical concern. The parents may be frightened at the prospect of the child dying at home and choose the security of the hospital; or, with sufficient preparation, they may want to keep him or her at home. The child may also express a preference in general terms about where he or she feels safe, or likes to be, even if not referring explicitly to death. All these factors must be taken into consideration. Whatever the setting, the parents' presence and contribution to the child's care and comfort are crucial.

The endpoint of the terminal phase is often marked by a turning inward on the part of the child, a decathecting from the external world. Cognitive and emotional horizons narrow, as all energy is needed simply for physical survival. A generalized irritability is not uncommon. The child may talk very little, and may even retreat from physical contact. Although such withdrawal is not universal, a certain degree of quietness is almost always evident. The child is pulling into him or herself, not away from others. If the parents understand this behavior as a normal and expectable precursor to death, they do not interpret it as rejection.[4] In certain instances, the therapist can play a crucial role in turning around the child's withdrawal and thus "returning" him or her to the parents.

Ricky had been exceedingly withdrawn over several days. He hardly talked, except to say, "I am in such discomfort," and lay with his back to everyone. The parents and therapist talked in Ricky's room about this dramatic change from his usual outgoing behavior. Ricky yelled: "Get out if you are going to talk." The therapist told him that it was important that he hear the discussion, even if he didn't feel like joining in. The therapist then began a monologue: "I wonder if you are just fed up with all this hospital stuff and treatments and that you still don't feel well.... I wonder if you feel kind of angry that nothing seems to be really helping you to feel much better...." After making several more statements about how he might possibly feel and how children in general feel, the therapist asked casually: "Do you think you feel a little like that?" Ricky said: "I guess so." The parents were startled and immediately pleased by his verbal acknowledgment. The therapist continued: "Kids sometimes feel mad ... mad at doctors, nurses, even their psychologist, and *even* their mother and father.... I wonder if you feel a little like that...." Ricky said clearly: "Yes." The therapist was then called out of the room for a few minutes. On her return, Ricky's mother reported that he had reached over and hugged her for the first time in days.

Withdrawal from the therapeutic relationship is also common. The child may not want to see the therapist or may be content simply for the therapist to stay with him or her, without much interaction. The child may even push away the therapeutic stuffed animal, previously an object of attachment. In many instances, the child seems to find it an unbearable reminder of playfulness and hope.

A week before her death, Jenny asked the therapist to bring Nutty the Squirrel to her hospital room. Jenny did not say anything when Nutty "arrived," but she placed him near her on the bed. By later that day, and continuing until her death, she refused to look at Nutty, or allow anyone to involve him in any form of communication.

A few days before Ricky died, his mother noticed him pushing his stuffed animals (his "sons and nephews") away from him on the bed. "Don't you want your sons near you?" she asked. Ricky replied: "I don't have any sons any more." These were the last words he spoke.[5]

The following description of the therapist's last three meetings with Jonathan provides a cameo of psychotherapy with the dying child. All the sessions took place in his hospital room. While it is rare for a child to remain so expressive into his or her final days, and for the therapist to have such access, the themes that emerged are universal.

First Session

The therapist brought Jonathan a colorful sticker from her office; he beamed on receiving it. She then began a monologue on how angry children get about being in the hospital, missing school, missing enjoyable activities, feeling sick, not having a good time. Jonathan listened, occasionally nodding in acknowledgment. His mother came into the room and told Jonathan that if he wished, she would take him to the therapist's office. Jonathan declined, but the offer led to a discussion of whether the therapist could bring her office to him. His first request was that "next time" the therapist bring her entire box of stickers so that he could choose one for himself. The therapist agreed and then slowly began to list Jonathan's "important" toys from the office (e.g., Walnut Bear, who was Jonathan's therapeutic stuffed animal; some small plastic animals; hospital figurines). "Should I bring Snoopy and Curious George also?" the therapist asked. "I told you to bring *everything*," retorted Jonathan. He then added magic markers and paper to the list but agreed that the therapist couldn't bring her desk. The therapist then told Jonathan that she would be leaving on vacation three days later. He did not react, except to ask whether she would send him a postcard. At this point, Jonathan's mother, who had left the room, rejoined the discussion.

anger about illness, missing out on normal childhood

importance of therapeutic space

child's assumption of therapeutic continuity

psychotherapy review; infusion of humor; small separation in context of ultimate separation, maintaining contact

She told Jonathan that she had just spoken to the director of his day camp and that Jonathan could go whenever he felt better; it didn't matter if he started late. (Jonathan had been looking forward to camp for months.) This information triggered the loudest most sustained protest that Jonathan had mounted in weeks: "IT'S NOT FAIR! I don't want to start camp late! If I have to start late, then everyone should start late. IT'S NOT FAIR!" After several minutes, Jonathan became quiet.

parent's involvement in therapeutic process

injustice of illness; fury at being different; loss of control over time

Second Session

The therapist came to Jonathan's room the next morning with a shopping bag full of toys from her office. As she took each object out of the bag, Jonathan watched carefully, without comment. He placed Walnut next to him on the bed. When the bag was empty, Jonathan said: "You forgot the little shells in the bottle." The therapist promised to bring them the next day. She then began to talk to Jonathan about Walnut's feelings. With the previous day's session in mind, the therapist described Walnut's being *angry* about being sick and missing out on things, pausing after each statement to ask: "Do you sometimes feel that way too?" Jonathan always nodded or said yes. When the therapist asked him if he could talk a little about that particular feeling, he would say simply: "I really can't say." Thus developed the pattern for the session: Jonathan would listen attentively and then acknowledge the feeling by saying: "Yes, but I really can't say." The therapist was talking quietly, almost hypnotically. Jonathan's gaze was riveted on her face. The therapist then

importance of fulfilling commitment to child

crucial role of therapeutic stuffed animal; acuity of memory of therapeutic space

permission for expression of anger

acknowledging the inexpressible

trust in therapeutic

moved on to *sad* feelings in her monologue: Walnut feeling so sad and alone about being sick and being in the hospital. She continued to question Jonathan about himself between each statement about Walnut. Jonathan began to pull Walnut closer toward him as she talked. The therapist then addressed feeling *scared:* "Walnut gets so scared sometimes . . . scared of feeling so sick . . . scared because he has never felt so sick before . . . scared because before, even when he was sick, he'd start to feel better, and now, not only does he not feel better, but maybe even worse . . . scared that something could happen to him . . . scared that maybe he could even die . . . scared about something bad and scary happening to him. Walnut gets the most scared when he is alone. . . . That's when he thinks sad and scary things. . . . Do you find that also?" "Sometimes," answered Jonathan, in the first break from his pattern of "Yes, but I really can't say." Throughout the "scared" segment, Jonathan continued to pull Walnut toward him, until he was resting in the crook of his arm. The therapist said: "Do you know that when Walnut was in my office, he was *crying?* He was just so lonely and scared." Jonathan looked at Walnut and turned his face toward him to see whether he was still crying. (By this point, Jonathan had been watching the therapist less and gazing directly at Walnut. It was almost as if he were hearing Walnut talk to him directly; he had lost track of the fact that it was the therapist's voice.) The therapist continued: "Walnut isn't crying any more, because he's visiting with you, and he

relationship; child feels alone in illness and dying, regardless of support

progression toward concept of dying and use of the word "dying"

significant change in response: more specific than general "yes"

identification with and empathy for therapeutic stuffed animal knows that you understand all his feelings." At this juncture, Jonathan asked: "Would it be all right for Walnut to stay with me tonight?" The therapist assented, and Jonathan fell asleep, clutching Walnut in his arm.

flexibility of rules

Third Session

As soon as the therapist entered the room, Jonathan asked whether she had remembered the shells. The therapist handed him the bottle. He scrutinized it, turning it around and around in his hand, examining it from every angle. He made no comment, just studied it silently. The therapist felt as if Jonathan were looking for some sort of sign or omen; as if one of the shells moved, it would mean "alive" for him. He looked at it for several minutes and then asked the therapist to put it on his tray. Walnut was propped up next to him on his pillow. (The nurses reported that when Jonathan had had a fever and chills earlier, he had asked for Walnut.) The therapist asked Jonathan how Walnut was feeling today. "Better," he answered. When asked what had made Walnut feel better, Jonathan replied: "Because he's with me." In response to Jonathan's request, the therapist agreed that Walnut and the bottle of shells could stay with him during her vacation. Jonathan asked whether he could telephone the therapist while she was away. The therapist wrote her number on an index card for him. Jonathan decided to decorate the card with a sticker from the sticker box that the therapist had brought. He sorted carefully through the se-

symbolic therapeutic object significant to child

hope for aliveness

companionship and comfort of therapeutic stuffed animal

maintenance of therapist's presence through therapeutic objects

planning for contact

lection, eventually choosing a teddy bear sticker, "because it's the same as the teddy bear sticker on your pager."

symbolic link of teddy bear sticker between child and therapist (telephone, pager)

Jonathan died peacefully two days later, with Walnut at his side.

❧ Epilogue

Thank you for giving me aliveness. *(Jonathan)*

Even when life itself cannot be guaranteed, psychotherapy can at least "give aliveness" to the child for however long that life may last.[1] The words of the children themselves lead the reader of this book into the child's experience of living between the light of hope and the shadow of threat. Through the extraordinary challenges posed by life-threatening illness, a precocious inner wisdom of life and its fragility emerges. Yet even in the struggle for survival, the spirit of childhood shines through. The children who are quoted are exceptionally articulate: they express what others feel. Their voices and images illuminate how illness is lived by the child, both physically and psychologically—in the external world and in the inner realm of symbolic meaning.

The essence of the therapist's task in working with the child with a life-threatening illness is captured in Colette's words: "Look long and hard at the things that please you, even longer and harder at what causes you pain."[2] To avert one's eyes is to lose the child, from a psychic point of view. While the child living the experience may need *not* to focus on the fulcrum of life and death, the therapist must be capable of the intensity of this gaze and able to sustain this intensity. At a profound intrapsychic level, the therapist's own strength comes from the ever present awareness of that fine line that separates living and dying. This knowledge becomes the containment of the psychotherapy. The unique psychological challenges for the therapist apply to a varying extent to all the caregivers involved with the child.

The therapist must be capable of witnessing and tolerating the anguish of threatened separation and loss. Inextricably linked with this psychic suffering are the harsh physical ravages of disease. To witness is not a passive process. In working with a child facing the possibility of death, the therapist must be able to enter the threat with the child, accompany him or her through the steps, while knowing that this may be a journey that they cannot complete together. There is a paradox intrinsic in the process: the therapist accompanies the child down a road toward what may be ultimate separation.

In order to allow the child full access to sadness and grief, the therapist must be able to contain and channel his or her own emotions. The therapist's personal loss history has impact on the psychotherapeutic work in the present. Memories of reactions to loss during childhood often provide pathways toward the child. Unresolved losses loom large in such encounters. The child has an acute sense of vision, through which the therapist's difficulties often become transparent. There is little space to hide. Thus, introspection must be the therapist's constant companion, with the attendant willingness to acknowledge vulnerability.

In the child's precarious life situation, the therapeutic role is highly specific: the therapist becomes an anchoring presence. While continuity is important in any psychotherapy, it is an absolute requisite in working with the seriously ill child. Within the context of the therapeutic relationship, the person of the therapist comes to embody the essence of that continuity. Availability and accessibility imply that consistent and abiding presence. The depth of the therapist's tenderness and commitment sustains the child in his or her confrontation with mortality.

For the child with a life-threatening illness, the family, and the caregivers, it is hope that infuses the pathway through the dark. The child reaches to catch and hold onto the light.

🌿 Appendix

Notes

✻ Appendix

My Life Is Feelings was conceptualized and written by Karen and the author over a three-month period of psychotherapy sessions. While the book served to integrate Karen's individual experience, it synthesizes many issues common to the child living with a life-threatening illness.

The photographs were retaken for better reproduction by Nancy R. Treves and Pamela M. Ryan.

My Life Is Feelings

Starring

Poly Polar Bear

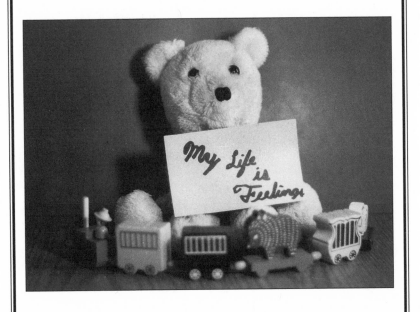

By:

Karen Josephson and Barbara M. Sourkes, Ph.D.

Photographs by:

Pamela M. Ryan, M.Ed., and Nancy R. Treves, M.Ed.

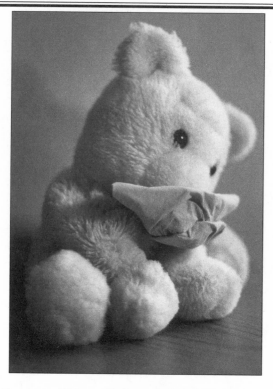

You have different feelings at different times, right? Well, so does Poly Polar Bear. Today Poly is crying. He is very worried because he knows that he has to have a finger stick or an IV. On other days, Poly Polar Bear might be frightened because of other things: all kinds of needles and tubes, blood tests, x-rays, scans, spinal taps, bone marrows, or even surgery. When Poly first started treatment, he was upset that he lost all his fur. Now, at last, his fur has grown back and he is not bald anymore.

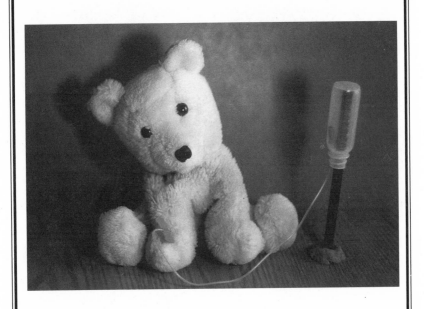

IVs for Poly are harder than they are for you, because if you look at Poly's paw, you can't tell where his veins are. Because Poly's paw is all furry!

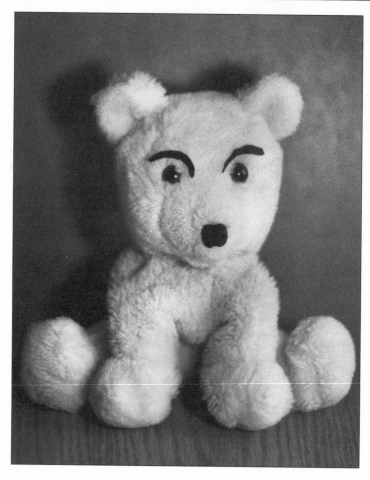

Poly is feeling MAD about everything today: family, school, treatment. "Why me?" he asks. That's the big question nowadays.

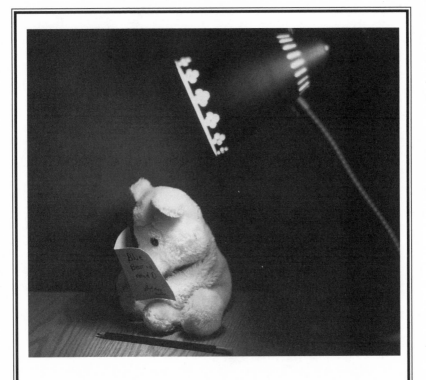

Poly is studying now. He misses school on days that he has to come to the clinic, or be in the hospital, or stay home when he doesn't feel well. Sometimes he feels sad and wishes that he could be in school with all his friends.

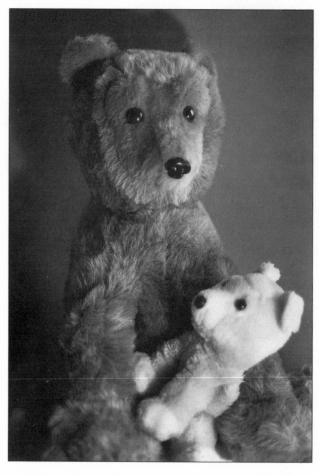

Poly loves to be loved, cuddled and held close. This
makes him feel happy and makes his hardships seem a
little easier.

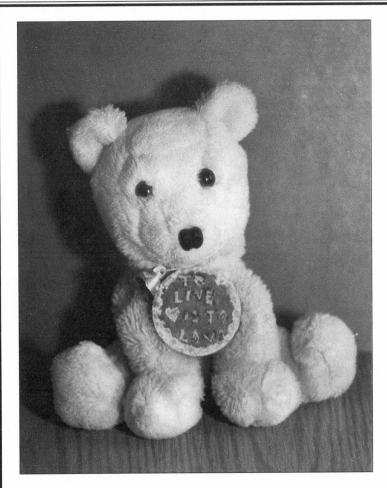

Poly Polar Bear has a very special wish: to be happy, healthy and to do well in school. He wears a button with his motto: TO LIVE IS TO LOVE.

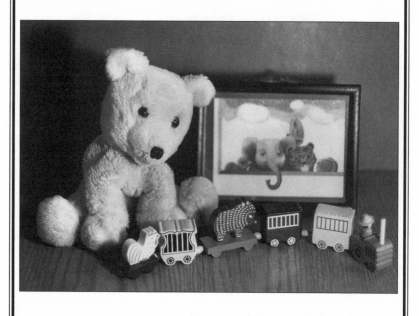

Now you have learned all about Poly Polar Bear and his feelings. Right now he is thinking about the future and what it beholds. Or maybe he is thinking about fun times in the past. He is very happy now as he plays with his train. Poly hopes that you have enjoyed his book, and he has something to say:

"Goodbye!"

Love
Poly Polar Bear

❧ Notes

CHAPTER I: PSYCHOTHERAPY

1. Barbara M. Sourkes, *The Deepening Shade: Psychological Aspects of Life-Threatening Illness* (Pittsburgh: University of Pittsburgh Press, 1982), p. 3.

2. Robert Coles, *The Spiritual Life of Children* (Boston: Houghton Mifflin, 1990), p. 101.

3. Lenore Terr, *Too Scared to Cry* (New York: Basic Books, 1990), p. 8.

4. Donald W. Winnicott, quoted in Madeleine Davis and David Wallbridge, *Boundary and Space: An Introduction to the Work of D. W. Winnicott* (New York: Brunner/Mazel, 1981), p. 44.

5. Ibid.

6. Ibid., p. 108.

7. Natalie Kusz, *Road Song* (New York: Farrar, Straus, Giroux, 1990), p. 95.

8. Donald W. Winnicott, *The Piggle: An Account of the Psychoanalytic Treatment of a Little Girl* (New York: International Universities Press, 1977), p. 47.

9. Jean Piaget and Bärbel Inhelder, *The Psychology of the Child* (New York: Basic Books, 1969).

10. Erik Erikson, *Childhood and Society* (New York: Norton, 1963).

11. Terr, *Too Scared to Cry*, p. 308.

12. See Sourkes, *Deepening Shade*, on framework issues in psychotherapy (e.g., time and space).

13. Margret Rey and H. A. Rey, *Curious George Goes to the Hospital* (Boston: Houghton Mifflin, 1966).

14. Davis and Wallbridge, *Boundary and Space*, p. 58.

15. Barbara M. Sourkes, "'All the Things I Don't Like About Having Leukemia': Children's Lists," in *Psychological Aspects of Childhood Cancer,* ed. J. Kellerman (Springfield: Charles C. Thomas, 1980), pp. 289–91.

16. The section on art techniques is adapted from Barbara M. Sourkes, "Truth to Life: Art Therapy with Pediatric Oncology Patients and Their Siblings," *Journal of Psychosocial Oncology* 9 (1991):81–96.

17. Susanne Fincher, *Creating Mandalas* (Boston: Shambhala Press, 1991).

18. Robert C. Burns and S. Harvard Kaufman, *Kinetic Family Drawings* (New York: Brunner/Mazel, 1970).

19. Terr, *Too Scared to Cry,* p. 307. "Therapist" has been substituted for "child psychiatrist" to be inclusive of all mental health professionals who work with children.

20. Sourkes, *Deepening Shade,* p. 12.

CHAPTER 2: ILLNESS AND TREATMENT

1. Barbara M. Sourkes, "The Child with a Life-Threatening Illness," in *Countertransference in Child and Adolescent Psychotherapy,* ed. J. Brandell (New York: Jason Aronson, 1992), p. 275.

2. Barbara M. Sourkes, "Truth to Life: Art Therapy with Pediatric Oncology Patients and Their Siblings," *Journal of Psychosocial Oncology* 9 (1991):86.

3. Barbara M. Sourkes, *The Deepening Shade: Psychological Aspects of Life-Threatening Illness* (Pittsburgh: University of Pittsburgh Press, 1982), p. 45.

4. The paragraphs on telling the diagnosis are adapted from Barbara M. Sourkes, "Psychologic Aspects of Leukemia and Other Hematologic Disorders," in *Hematology of Infancy and Childhood,* ed. D. G. Nathan and F. Oski, 4th ed. (Philadelphia: W. B. Saunders, 1992), pp. 1754–68.

5. Mark A. Chesler, Jan Paris, and Oscar A. Barbarin, "Telling the Child with Cancer: Parental Choices to Share Information with Ill Children," *Journal of Pediatric Psychology* 11 (1986):514.

6. Marie-Claude Charest and Suzanne Douesnard, "La verité sort de la bouche des enfants," *P.R.I.S.M.E.* 2 (1992):473.

7. Sourkes, "Truth to Life," p. 89.

8. Sourkes, "Psychologic Aspects," p. 1756.

9. Madeleine Davis and David Wallbridge, *Boundary and Space: An Introduction to the Work of D. W. Winnicott* (New York: Brunner/Mazel, 1981), p. 38.

10. See the appendix.

11. Natalie Kusz, *Road Song* (New York: Farrar, Straus, Giroux, 1990), pp. 108, 102.

12. They were first published in Sourkes, "Truth to Life," p. 91.

13. Sourkes, "Child with a Life-Threatening Illness," p. 282.

14. Sourkes, "Truth to Life," p. 93.

15. Winnicott, quoted in Davis and Wallbridge, *Boundary and Space,* p. 36.

16. Kusz, *Road Song,* p. 110.

17. The description of the bone marrow transplantation procedure is adapted from Sourkes, "Psychologic Aspects."

18. Sourkes, "Child with a Life-Threatening Illness," p. 281.

19. The clinical work with K and S was done by Nancy R. Treves, under the supervision of the author.

20. The section on elective cessation of treatment is adapted from Sourkes, *Deepening Shade.*

21. Ibid., p. 62.

22. Ibid., p. 61.

CHAPTER 3: IMPACT ON NORMAL LIFE

1. Lenore Terr, *Too Scared to Cry* (New York: Basic Books, 1990), p. 289.

2. Barbara M. Sourkes, "The Child with a Life-Threatening Illness," in *Countertransference in Child and Adolescent Psychotherapy,* ed. J. Brandell (New York: Jason Aronson, 1992), p. 275.

3. Terr, *Too Scared to Cry,* p. 49.

4. Douglas S. Rait and Jimmie C. B. Holland, "Pediatric Cancer: Psychosocial Issues and Approaches," in *Mediguide to Oncology* 6 (1986):4.

5. Murray Bowen, "Family Reaction to Death," in *Family Therapy,* ed. P. J. Guerin (New York: Gardner, 1976), p. 339.

6. On the psychological issues faced by siblings, see Barbara M. Sourkes, "Siblings of the Pediatric Cancer Patient," in *Psychological Aspects of Childhood Cancer,* ed. J. Kellerman (Springfield: Charles C. Thomas, 1980), pp. 47–69. This chapter was reprinted in slightly different form in

"Siblings of the Child with a Life-Threatening Illness," *Journal of Children in Contemporary Society* 19 (1987):159–184.

7. Erik Erikson, *Childhood and Society* (New York: Norton, (1963).

8. Kusz, *Too Scared to Cry*, p. 98.

CHAPTER 4: FACETS OF AWARENESS

1. See Myra Bluebond-Langner's conceptualization of stages of awareness in *The Private Worlds of Dying Children* (Princeton, N.J.: Princeton University Press, 1978).

2. Barbara M. Sourkes, *The Deepening Shade: Psychological Aspects of Life-Threatening Illness* (Pittsburgh: University of Pittsburgh Press, 1982), p. 28.

3. Natalie Kusz, *Road Song* (New York: Farrar, Straus, Giroux, 1990), p. 100.

4. Sourkes, *Deepening Shade*, p. 16.

5. Barbara M. Sourkes, "The Child with a Life-Threatening Illness," in *Countertransference in Child and Adolescent Psychotherapy*, ed. J. Brandell (New York: Jason Aronson, 1992), p. 277.

6. Ibid., p. 273.

7. Kusz, *Too Scared to Cry*, p. 100.

8. Sourkes, *Deepening Shade*, p. 18.

9. Donald W. Winnicott, *Therapeutic Consultations in Child Psychiatry* (New York: Basic Books, 1971), p. 115.

10. Sourkes, *Deepening Shade*, p. 70.

11. Winnicott, *Therapeutic Consultations*, p. 32.

12. Joyce Johnson, "The Children's Wing," in *Prize Stories: O. Henry Awards* (New York: Doubleday, 1987), p. 16.

13. Robert Coles, *The Spiritual Life of Children* (Boston: Houghton Mifflin, 1990), p. 101.

14. Sourkes, *Deepening Shade*, p. 23.

15. Drawing contributed by Nancy R. Treves.

CHAPTER 5: ANTICIPATORY GRIEF

1. Barbara M. Sourkes, *The Deepening Shade: Psychological Aspects of Life-Threatening Illness* (Pittsburgh: University of Pittsburgh Press, 1982), p. 37.

2. See ibid. for a more detailed discussion of the three axes of loss.

3. Erik Erikson, *Childhood and Society* (New York: Norton, (1963).

4. C. Knight Aldrich, "Some Dynamics of Anticipatory Grief," in *Anticipatory Grief,* ed. B. Schoenberg et al. (New York: Columbia University Press, 1974), p. 4.

5. Barbara M. Sourkes, "Siblings of the Pediatric Cancer Patient," in *Psychological Aspects of Childhood Cancer,* ed. J. Kellerman (Springfield: Charles C. Thomas, 1987), p. 63.

6. Drawing contributed by the family of Jonathan (Jay) Hager.

7. Barbara M. Sourkes, "The Child with a Life-Threatening Illness," in *Countertransference in Child and Adolescent Psychotherapy,* ed. J. Brandell (New York: Jason Aronson, 1992), p. 279.

8. Ibid.

9. Ibid., p. 271.

CHAPTER 6: THE DYING CHILD

1. Adapted from Barbara M. Sourkes, *The Deepening Shade: Psychological Aspects of Life-Threatening Illness* (Pittsburgh: University of Pittsburgh Press, 1982), and "Psychologic Aspects of Leukemia and Other Hematologic Disorders," in *Hematology of Infancy and Childhood,* ed. D. G. Nathan and F. Oski, 4th ed. (Philadelphia: W. B. Saunders, 1992).

2. Sourkes, *Deepening Shade,* p. 83.

3. Ibid.

4. Sourkes, "Psychologic Aspects," p. 1756.

5. Sourkes, *Deepening Shade,* p. 84.

EPILOGUE

1. Part of the epilogue is adapted from Barbara M. Sourkes, "The Child with a Life-Threatening Illness," in *Countertransference in Child and Adolescent Psychotherapy,* ed. J. Brandell (New York: Jason Aronson, 1992). It is reprinted with permission.

2. Colette, *Lettres au petit corsaire* (Paris: Flammarion, 1963).